Praise for The Lunchbox Effect

As a Paediatric Endocrinologist, Diabetologist and Child Obesity Expert, I witness first-hand the devastating effect processed food can have on children's physical and mental health and behaviour which all impact on a child fulfilling their potential in life.

There has never been a more pressing time in the history of Children's Health in Australia with more children suffering from obesity and type 2 diabetes. We simply have to start taking action now. The Lunchbox Effect shines a light on how processed foods found in lunchboxes is having an impact on the health and education of Australian children. Belinda takes a sensible and practical approach to offering parents solutions to easily identify what's in lunchbox foods and simple swaps to make lunchboxes more nutritious.

Dr Gary Leong

Paediatric Endocrinologist, Diabetologist and Child Obesity Expert and Author of "Ride to Life a no-nonsense program to breaking your family's cycle of obesity"

Wow! Thank you Belinda. As a teacher, this book says everything I have wanted to say about how lunchboxes are affecting classrooms but can't because of fear of backlash from parents and the system. It is time for parents, teachers and the Government to stand together for Children's Health. Action to address the food in school lunchboxes needs to be taken.

Pauline Beal

Teacher of 20 years

I first met Belinda when she gave evidence to the 2018 Senate Select Committee into The Obesity Epidemic. I was inspired by her passion and understanding of the impact food is having at a grass roots level - in homes and at schools - around Australia. From her involvement with the Committee, Belinda quickly recognised creating political change at a national level takes considerable time. Her belief that we can't wait for years for action to take place, led her to write her book The Lunchbox Effect. The book raises much needed awareness about what is in common lunchbox foods and how these foods are affecting health, academic results and waste. The Lunchbox Effect is a captivating read and a real call to parents, teachers, the school system and government to start taking action now. Politicians, especially those in Ministries of Health and Education need to read this book.

Former Senator The Honourable **Lisa Singh**

Belinda has worked so hard over the last few years, her passion and dedication to children's health is commendable. The Lunchbox Effect, is a compelling read for parents, teachers and those in positions of influence in children's lives. Belinda explores the impact of children's lunchboxes in classrooms and how schools and busy parents are both trying to give children the best chance to succeed in their learning.

Louise Stone

Principal for 8 years of 2 schools, and teacher for 30 years

The Lunchbox Effect tells an alarming story of how the normalisation of processed food is affecting Children's Health, the education system and our environment. The book does not shy away from industry, instead it exposes what's in common lunchbox foods with the express aim of helping parents make better choices for their children.

Georgia Harding

Naturopath

I first met Bel about 3 years ago. At the time, it's safe to say my two sons and myself were not in great health. Hearing Bel talk about what's in the food we were eating totally changed our lives. We began turning packets over and reading what was in the food. Our health improved dramatically. More importantly, Bel's messages have stuck. What I love about The Lunchbox Effect is Bel is still spreading the same simple messages. I know with this book, Bel is going to change lives, just like how she changed ours.

Lori

Mum of 2 healthy boys

As a mum of 5 children, all who are sensitive to additives and preservatives, I love that The Lunchbox Effect is highlighting the impacts these ingredients can have on some children. My kids ask for packet foods because their friends are eating them and it is hard as a mum to stand my ground and say no but I have too because I know what this food does to them. Thank you Belinda for raising awareness about what's in these foods and giving me the courage to make a stand for my children's health.

Amanda

Mother of 5

Being born in the 1950', eating wholefoods was just the way everyone ate, it wasn't a buzz word. Today, society is largely disconnected from food - how it's grown, produced and the need to eat for health are not top of mind. In writing The Lunchbox Effect, Belinda has exposed how significant this disconnection with our food has become in school lunchboxes. Belinda takes a bold stance by highlighting the problems this is creating for Children's Health, the education system and the planet. I particularly love how she is calling on parents to cook more at home, but importantly for the Government to return cooking to the school system.

Jude Blereau

Whole and Natural Foods Chef, Award-Winning Author, Speaker and Cooking Teacher

Any action to keep junk food out of schools and to introduce children to food that will keep them happy, healthy and ready to learn is a really good idea! The Lunchbox Effect is a call to the Australian Government to take action. We also urge the Australian government to follow the UK's lead by introducing standards for school food and lunch boxes, to help schools and parents to lay the foundations for a lifetime of good food, health and happiness.

Stephanie Wood

Founder/CEO, School Food Matters

The Lunchbox Effect is a compelling book sharing how far Australian lunchboxes have strayed from nourishing children's bodies and brains. It really highlights the importance of the work both The Good Foundation and The Root Cause do in helping Australian transform their eating habits. In this book, Belinda provides parents with eye opening information about what's in common lunchbox packets and tips on simple swaps to make lunches more nutritious. A must read for every parent with school aged children.

Siobhan Boyle

CEO of The Good Foundation. The Good Foundation proudly presents Jamie's Ministry of Food and Jamie's Learn Your Fruit and Vegetables Programs in Australia.

the
lunchbox
effect

How today's lunchbox foods are impacting
your child's learning, behaviour and health,
and what you can do about it.

BELINDA SMITH

Editor: Dannielle Line
Proofread: Carolyn De Ridder
Interior design: Ida Jansson

National Library of Australia Cataloguing-in-Publication data:
The Lunchbox Effect/ Belinda Smith
Non Fiction/Nutrition

ISBN: 978-0-6487624-5-4 (sc)
ISBN: 978-0-6487624-6-1 (e)

About the Author

BELINDA SMITH

Belinda Smith, co-founder of The Root Cause, is one of Australia's leading independent voices on children's health, and an advocate for real food in schools. Belinda is also a mum, a health coach, and the creator of The Mad Food Science Incursion and The Children's Health Program, The 5 Minute Healthy Lunchbox System, and Kids Food Quest.

After travelling Australia for two and a half years visiting over 90 schools and educating more than 20,000 children, teachers and parents, Belinda truly understands what is going on in our school system when it comes to food.

Bel has been dubbed "The Lunchbox Vigilante" by Channel 7 Sunrise, and appears regularly in national and regional TV, radio and press. Bel was mentioned in Federal Parliament for the work she has been doing across Australia with The Root Cause.

Bel's vision is to create a generation of healthy, food-literate children who choose real food every day.

Dedication

I dedicate this book to my children, Indrani and Rilien. My love for you knows no bounds, and I will always prioritise your health over convenience. I want you both to grow up in a world where you eat real food every day without feeling abnormal. I want you to grow up in a world where you and your friends live a long life free from chronic illness. To Israel, my amazing husband, thank you for giving me the reason to look at what we were eating, that changed the course of direction of our family's health. I thank you for being right by my side, believing in me and my passion to take on this problem of children's health.

Out of love and respect, we dedicate this book to all parents and teachers.

The Root Cause exists for you. Our vision is to create a generation of healthy, food literate children who choose real food every day, enabling them to be better learners, more successful students, and go on to help build stronger, healthier, more sustainable communities. We want to create a world where it is easier for parents to get their children to eat more fruits and vegetables. We want to create a world where teachers spend more time teaching with less stress. With your help, we know we can do this. Thank you!

Every child deserves the right to live their life to their full potential, without chronic illness.

Acknowledgements

The publication of this book has only been made possible with the generous contributions of many amazing people and organisations.

I'd like to express my deepest thanks to everyone who has supported and encouraged me throughout this process. I am forever grateful for your support in helping me bring the vision of this book to life, and I'm immensely proud of what we've produced together. (And if I have accidentally omitted anyone from this list, please accept my apology and my gratitude, and let me know so I can put your name in the next edition!)

In particular, I'd like to thank the beautiful individuals and companies listed below who contributed time and energy to this project, by writing chapters, compiling product data, analysing and reviewing that data, and finally shaping my words and ideas into the beautiful book you're reading now. Thank you.

- My amazing family – Israel, Indrani and Rilien.
- Kate Tonkin, our WA based Certified Instructor for gifting us a book title that says exactly what we wanted it to say.
- Our incredibly passionate Certified Instructors past and present, and especially those who helped with the data collection and proofreading: Gemma McPhee, Karen Wong, Kate Tonkin, Kirsty Bear, Lauren Martin, Lauren Symes, Natasha Dawson, Tanya Pichler, Veronica Pasfield and Victoria Byrnes.

- Rob Dallimore, Deborah Van Wyk and the amazing marketing team at Worldwide – our long-term National Partner – for believing in The Root Cause at the very beginning and supporting us every step of the way.
- Loren Downing and Rob Bartlett from Sync Or Swim (SOS) – our data partner – for pulling together and making sense of the mountains of data from the product reviews in this book.
- Dr Charlotte Middleton – Integrative GP, specialising in Maternity, Paediatric, Nutritional and Environmental Medicine, who isn't afraid to talk about the elephant in the room – food and the impacts on children's health.
- Susan Hilliar – One of the bravest and strongest Principals I have met to date.
- Madison Hille - Accredited Practising Dietitian (APD), BNutDietet (Hons) for completing the final quality review of the individual products reviewed in this book.
- Jo Atkinson - Nutritional Medicine Practitioner BHSc (Nut Med) for her incredible ability to make complex information about nutritional requirements seem easy.
- Francine Bell – Additive Free Food Coach and Consultant for shining the light on additives and preservatives in a way that gets us thinking.
- Karen McDermott – our Publisher who helped bring this book into the world.
- Dannielle Line – our Editor who tirelessly kept up with all the changes I kept making to the book.
- Ida Jansson – our Designer who crafted words, tables, fonts and quotes into a gorgeous interior design.
- May Phan – for the most wonderful cover design that kept me motivated to finish writing this book
- Liz & Anthony Phillips, Dr Tony Pennells & Raj Kale – for your generosity, support and mentoring.

Contents

Disclaimer

This book is intended for educational purposes and for general information only. I do not intend it to provide scientific, medical or health advice for your family. I intend the book to enable readers to make their own choices about which processed and pre-packaged foods best suit their family and individual children's needs. The author and contributors are in no way responsible for, or liable for, any losses, damage or harm which may result because of the use of information in this guide. Your own research is an essential component of all that is exposed in this book. Speak to your own medical or health practitioner for specific advice regarding your own family.

I have collated this book through my personal experiences and research, with the assistance of thirteen contributors. I do not intend the information in this book to constitute scientific or medical advice. I intend this book to be a comprehensive guide to the wide variety of foods being marketed and eaten as school lunchbox food. Any omission of a product does not indicate the product is not a lunchbox food or doesn't warrant asking the question of "What's In My Food?" I do not intend to cover all information about the products included in the book. The author and the contributors to this book have made every effort to ensure the information is accurate and current as at the date the information was researched (Dec 2018 – Feb 2019).

The author and contributors all acknowledge there is a place in today's world for processed, packaged food and recommend readers always consciously choose packaged food only after asking "What's In

My Food?" The author and contributors do not endorse, recommend or promote any one product over another. Many references available in the public domain were consulted and cross-referenced in collating the information in this book. The author and the contributors do not guarantee the accuracy of the information obtained from these references and denies liability for the accuracy of that information. It is the reader's responsibility to validate the accuracy of the information most relevant to them.

The author understands statistics and product formulations may change from time to time and welcomes any updates from any person, organisation or product manufacturer for any product included in this book. This way any omissions, errors or changes in the ingredients and nutritional information can be corrected and update in future editions. Updates will be made to the book's Online Product Companion website app as soon as practically possible.

Foreword

The Lunchbox Effect from Belinda Smith and The Root Cause team couldn't have come at a better time. The World Health Organisation (WHO) has now labelled childhood obesity as one of the most serious public health issues of the 21st century. In Australia, 1 in 4 children are now overweight or obese. Children who are obese are more likely to have high blood pressure, high cholesterol, impaired glucose tolerance, insulin resistance, type 2 diabetes, breathing problems such as asthma and sleep apnoea, joint problems and musculoskeletal discomfort, fatty liver, gallstones and heartburn. We also know we can relate childhood obesity to psychological problems such as anxiety and depression, low self-esteem and social problems such as bullying and stigma.

Overweight and obese children typically grow into overweight and obese adults, who are susceptible to chronic complaints such as diabetes, cardiovascular disease, arthritis, depression and cancer. These diseases place considerable burdens on the individual, the family, the national health systems and the Australian economy.

There is even talk now that for the first time ever in history, children may live shorter lives than their parents. Or if they do live longer, they will have more years of poor quality health than their parents, due to these chronic illnesses.

As an Integrative GP, specialising in nutritional and environmental medicine, I've become increasingly concerned with the number of overweight or obese children I see in my daily practice. But it's not just obesity that is the concern here. I am also seeing an increasing number of children with mental health issues, behavioural issues and learning difficulties. Many parents are reporting problems at school and are at a loss as to what they can do.

While all these issues (including obesity) will be multifactorial in origin, I am absolutely convinced (with the science and research to back me), what children put in their mouth, is a major causative factor. Processed and packaged foods full of sugar, trans fats, salt, preservatives and additives are known to adversely affect our children in every way possible. Additives alone have been shown to cause symptoms ranging from poor attention and concentration, hyperactivity and anxiety to skin rashes, headaches and recurrent respiratory illnesses.

Sugar is a particularly hot topic now, and understandably so. 75% of all packaged foods contain added sugar, so most children are having much more than their recommended quota of under 4-6 teaspoons (16-24g) of added sugar per day. I cannot emphasise the implications of excess sugar intake enough with tooth decay, hyperactivity, weakened immunity and nutritional deficiencies—just a few of the common symptoms I see.

I am all too aware eating healthily can be a challenge at times. As a working mum with two small children myself, stressed and time poor, the allure and convenience of packaged food is hard to resist. And the constant mixed messages we receive about what is, and is not healthy, makes packing your child's lunch box all the more complex.

Reading the product labels and understanding the ingredients is not always easy and, let's face it, who has the time anyway?

The Lunchbox Effect with its comprehensive guide to what's in lunchbox packet foods can help, by taking the guesswork out of reading labels. Literacy in reading labels is a vital skill for all consumers and with it comes the feeling of confidence when choosing packaged foods, that we're still making a smart choice for our family.

Changing what we eat and how we feed our family doesn't have to be hard. And it doesn't have to be all or nothing. Even small changes in children's lunchboxes can have a profound impact. Just including more fruits and vegetables and reducing processed, packaged foods (i.e. from two packets to one), will produce many health benefits. When you include packaged food, ask what's in it and make the healthiest possible choice for your child.

Now more than ever, we need organisations like The Root Cause. Their work improving the health of children by empowering them to make better food choices - and now this book exposing what's in lunchbox packet foods - goes a long way to reducing the devastating impact processed foods are having on the lives of our children.

Dr Charlotte Middleton
BMBS, Dip CH, FRACGP

A Dietician's Perspective

Dietitian Madison Hille completed the quality review of the product data we have included in this book. She shares her views:

The content of a child's lunchbox is not just food; it's the food that has to provide them with the energy to get through an entire day of learning, playing and after school activities. When looking at it like this, the food in a child's lunchbox is perhaps the most important food they consume in a day. Yet, a large portion of Australian school lunchboxes are made up of what we call 'discretionary foods'. Discretionary foods do not fit into the Five Food Groups because they are not necessary for a healthy diet and are too high in saturated fat and/or added sugars, added salt and low in fibre.

Often we think we are doing the right thing by filling kids lunchboxes with muesli bars, savoury crackers, juice, fruit cups etc. but reality is many of these foods are actually classified as discretionary foods. The last AIHW report on nutrition across life stages shows on average, primary aged children are eating 4.8 to 6.2 serves of discretionary foods a day. It's important to note that the recommended number of serves per day is 0 to 2. We also know that nearly 40% of energy is coming from discretionary foods in school-aged children.

As well as contributing to excessive energy, saturated fat, sugar and salt consumption, discretionary foods can take the place of other more nutritious foods. The AIHW report also shows that Australian kids are not eating enough fruit, vegetables, wholegrain cereal foods or dairy foods. In fact, just one in 17 Aussie children are eating the recommended number of serves of both fruit and vegetables.

Consuming discretionary foods occasionally or in moderation is all part of a balanced diet, however Australian school children are consuming far more than that of a balanced diet. The negative impacts of excessive discretionary food consumption go far beyond weight gain and the increased the risk of obesity. Poor oral health, micronutrient deficiencies, gastrointestinal issues as a result of poor fibre intake and even mental health issues can all result from excessive discretionary food intake. More recent studies have shown that a diet high in discretionary foods can negatively impact on academic performance and behaviour at school. A diet high in discretionary food doesn't provide children with adequate energy to get them through their busy days, often leaving them burnout.

We need to move away from the convenience foods packed with saturated fat, sugar and salt and move towards wholefoods rich in nutrients. Children should be actively involved in their lunch preparation. In doing so, they will be much more likely to eat the food and they will be learning about the importance of nutritious foods.

Madison Hille
Accredited Practising Dietitian (APD), BNutDietet (Hons)

Introduction /
About This Book

I wrote this book to raise awareness about what's in lunchbox packet foods and the potential effects of the different ingredients they contain. It's designed to help busy parents to make better food choices for lunchbox food and to help you easily see what's in the most common lunchbox packets. This information will help you consciously choose what packets, if any, you want to send with your children to school.

Please remember, this is coming from a place of love for all children and respect for you as a parent. It's not about saying packet foods are evil. We realise in a busy world, there's a place and need for them. Each of the people who contributed to this book have some packets in our pantries. As we unveil the information, I want you to know, there is no judgement about what you've been packing in your child's lunchbox. My desire is to be of service. Every single mum who is a contributor to this book is like me. We did not know this information until someone else pointed it out to us or we each started to research to solve a health challenge for ourselves or a loved one. The information we each uncovered led us to change the food we eat. From the changes we've each made, we've reaped the rewards seeing positive impacts on our children's health and behaviour, or even our own health. Our hope is that the findings we share through this book, "The Lunchbox Effect" may be an inspiration to you.

Independent Voices

This book gives you an independent picture of what's in the most common lunchbox packet foods. It has been carefully curated by a group of passionate mums who are totally independent. We are not funded by any external organisation, backed by government, or lobbying for a particular industry group or corporate vested interest. The only vested interest we have is to make sure our children, and yours, grow up in a world where they choose real food every day as their normal food. We believe in the power of parents. As parents, we don't have to wait for rules or government policy on what to feed our families. We can start feeding our children and families food that helps their bodies and brains grow and develop in a healthy way.

As a busy parent who learned the hard way about the connection between food and the impact it was having on my family, I want to make it easy for you. I share our story and the information in this book with the hope it will make your life easier as a parent and create a healthier generation of children too. In this book, busy parents will learn the effects the food packed in children's lunchboxes can have on a child's learning, behaviour and health. You'll also get some great tips on steps you can take to make better food choices for your children and how to have conversations with them about food that bring them along for the ride. In addition, at your fingertips will be a quick look guide including the ingredients of over 480 common lunchbox packet foods, including breads and wraps.

As we begin right here, right now, I want you to know wherever you are at is totally perfect. Remember, we only ever make choices with the knowledge we have available to us any given time, and the choices we make are the best we are capable of at that time. Please use the information in this book to look forward. What choices can you now make with this new knowledge?

Wherever you are at is totally perfect!

Each of us contributing to this book believed, prior to embarking on this project, we were well-educated about what's in our food. However, having taken the time to read every packet label on over 480 common lunchbox packets has shown us otherwise. We struggled to comprehend what some of these ingredients were. We lost track of the number of hours of research we've put into creating this information for you. I can share it took me personally over ten hours to photograph the products alone.

Several times I was ready to give up on this book. Many times it seemed too hard, too big. I was in utter shock and often overwhelmed at the sheer volume of products on the supermarket shelves. It is no wonder these products have become "normal" food in lunchboxes. Wherever I turned in the aisles, there were products telling me they are: "lunchbox friendly", "perfect for lunchboxes" and so on.

Many times I'd become momentarily overwhelmed, and my hubby would remind me this is the reason this book needs to be out in the world. To help make it less confusing for others. To make it easy for parents to have the knowledge so they can make informed decisions for themselves and the health of their family.

We have done our absolute best in collating the information in this book. On a project this size, with the complexities of the number of ingredients in these foods, there is potential for inaccuracies. In addition, food manufacturers do from time to time change the formulation of their products. So we've based the information contained in this document on the ingredients and Nutrition Information Panel available for sale December 2018 and February 2019. In assessing the potential effects of the additives and preservatives we have used "The Chemical Maze app", the Food Intolerance Network (fedup.com.au) and Additive Free Kids (additivefreekids.com.au). These are fantastic resources and we encourage you to do your own research too. The Additive Alert book by Julie Eady is a wonderful and eye opening read. You will also find a load of information from Additive Free Lifestyle too (additivefreelifestyle.com).

Using this Book

While I'm sure you are super keen to jump straight to the Lunchbox Product Reference section to check what's in your lunchbox packet foods, I strongly suggest you read the entire book in order to give you context as to why we parents need to take a stand for our own children's health. The chapters build on each other to give you a deeper knowledge about all the issues. This knowledge will give you strength to continue standing for your own children's health even whilst it seems you may be swimming against the tide of what others are doing.

Throughout this book, you will also find references to additional materials I have developed to help you. We have built a special website to house all these materials for you in one spot.

Grab your FREE Bonuses for The Lunchbox Effect:
http://thelunchboxeffect.com/bonuses

You may also wish to purchase the Online Product Companion that accompanies this book.

The Online Product Companion is a smartphone-optimised

website app with a fully-searchable database of all the 480+ products listed in the Lunchbox Product Reference section of this book. It includes full colour photographs, more detailed images of each product (such as Ingredients and Nutritional Information Panel), and more comprehensive data tables for each product. It allows you to search a product quickly and easily at your fingertips on your phone or tablet.

Purchase The Lunchbox Effect
Online Product Companion:
http://thelunchboxeffect.com/opc

Long Term Change Starts with Simple Nudges

Anything that is hard doesn't stick. That's why diets rarely work long-term. They feel like hard work or they leave you feeling like you're being deprived. This book is not about throwing everything out and starting from scratch. It's not about saying don't buy any more packet foods. It's about becoming more conscious and smarter with what we do buy.

It's about making small nudges in what
you currently do, so new choices become a way of life.

Here are some simple nudges to start with:
- Pack more fruits and vegetables in lunchboxes.
- If you normally send your child to school with two packets, start by sending them off with one packet and adding in more fruits and vegetables (if three packets, send two etc). Over time keep changing this to maybe sending one every second day. Make the changes gradually so it's easier for everyone.

- Choose the plain variety of packets rather than the flavoured packets.
- Pack a filling main lunch (Chapter 13 will help with this).
- Send water to school. Keep the other drinks for home if you want the kids to have them.

Making a conscious choice to choose health
over convenience is where it starts.

We hope this book helps you understand the effect your child's lunchbox can have on their health, behaviour, mood, concentration, learning ability and sleeping habits. We hope it gives you the "why"for making changes, starting now.

I sincerely thank you for your interest in this book and I encourage you to join us in Standing for Children's Health.

Much love & wellness,
Belinda Smith

PART 1:

How did we get here?

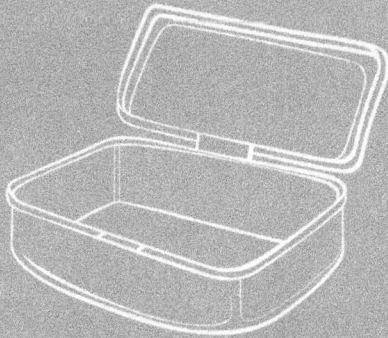

Chapter 1
Our Journey to Health

I am a mum who nine years ago thought I was doing a great job at feeding my family. I cooked at home every night and sent my daughter off to school with a packed lunch of a sandwich, a piece of fruit and a few different lunchbox packet foods. I didn't think twice about what was in those packet foods as I bought many of them from the health food aisle in the supermarket. My daughter started school when our second child, our son, was about five months old. I was doing my best to keep up with the demands of a new baby and keep my daughter well-fed at school.

It was at this time my husband, Israel, was diagnosed with post-natal depression, and started getting professional help for his mental health. Israel wanted to explore other treatment options rather than medication as the first option, believing that there must be some underlying issue causing his depression.

With the guidance of Israel's psychologist, we looked at his sleep, exercise and what he was eating. I read everything I could about the impacts of food on mental health. This is when I discovered the connection between food and how it makes us feel. To my shock and dismay, I also discovered the food I'd been packing in my daughter's lunchbox had been affecting her health, temperament, and ability to concentrate and learn—without me even realising it.

Changing What We Ate

Motivated mostly by getting my husband's mental state back to normal, I focused my energy on feeding our family real foods. We ate lots of fresh raw vegetables every day, small amounts of fruit and good quality meats. I eliminated most foods that came in a packet and if I bought packet food, it was only after scrutinising what the ingredients were. Essentially, I stopped using any packaged food that had ingredients I didn't recognise. We even eliminated most gluten from our diet after learning that for some people it can be a major contributor to mental illnesses such as depression or anxiety.

In a matter of weeks, Israel said he felt a fog had lifted. Whilst he was still suffering depression, his symptoms had substantially improved. What also surprised us was the change in our daughter's behaviour. Back then our volatile five-year-old girl could be happily playing and then at the drop of a hat, she was crying. We'd accepted this was who she was, and this was how our lives would be as parents. However, as we started to eat more real food and reducing processed foods, her volatility levelled out. Rarely were there moments of unexplained crying. Her temperament settled. The blue rings she had under her eyes that we'd accepted as part of her also disappeared.

Changing what we ate took a bit of effort but parenting our daughter became easier.

Learning to Ask: "What's In My Food?"

The most significant learning for Israel and myself was to ask ONE simple question: "What's In My Food?"

We discovered there were many ingredients in our food that were not real. Ingredients created using food science and technology in a chemistry lab, then made in a factory by combining it with other ingredients. Once combinations of ingredients are perfected, they're mass produced in a factory and become the products we buy from the supermarket. Many of these ingredients, namely additives, have been linked to health conditions such as depression, anxiety, behaviour issues, asthma, sleep disturbance and more. I also discovered many of the jars, sachets, pouches and packets I'd been using in my daily cooking were laced with sugar, salts, fats and flavour enhancers. I added up how much sugar, salt, fat, flavour enhancers were in the different foods we were eating in a day. I realised we were consuming excessively more than the recommended amounts of these ingredients for good health.

I realised the cooking at home I was doing was in fact not cooking from scratch at all, and the lunch I was packing was not great either.

I discovered I was cooking with **some** real food ingredients, but to add flavour and taste, I was mixing in ingredients made in a chemistry lab and factory. Uncovering this information on additives helped me realise those convenient packets I was sending our daughter to school with were a chemical concoction of ingredients. These ingredients were doing precious little to help her body or brain in its growth and development. I discovered I was sending her body on a roller coaster ride on the inside. Essentially, the packaged and convenient foods were creating energy highs followed by energy crashes. Consistently and repeatedly. Doing this to a body every day that is trying to grow and develop is not great nor helpful. Was it any wonder she was having trouble concentrating at school and at home and that she had volatile behaviour?

My research into ingredients in packaged food taught me a significant amount of the foods we ate were "discretionary". These foods are not part of the five food groups our bodies require for health. They are foods that are only recommended to be eaten sometimes and in small amounts. Not daily and in multiple quantities. When I was growing up, my mum would have called many of these foods "junk foods". I am not sure why I, as a parent, didn't think of these foods as "junk foods" or why I thought my daughter needed them every day in her lunchbox. In my defence, I have to remember, I was a full time working mother. I shopped according to what was presented to me in catalogues, on TV and on display at the supermarkets, especially those items on sale. What other mums in my circle of friends were doing for their kids directly influenced me. If they were having success in getting their children to eat certain foods, then I would try it too.

A Much Bigger Problem

The realisation of what was in the food we were eating and how it could impact our mental and physical health, gave me the impetus to study and learn more. I learnt not just about food, but what was and is still happening to the health of children in Australia (and around the world).

Here's what I now know to be true.

"Food can nourish, energise, protect and support our bodies, or it can bring us down."

SHERRY STRONG,
AUTHOR OF *RETURN TO FOOD: THE LIFE CHANGING ANTI-DIET*

We all understand how food gives us nourishment and energy, but it's the "bringing us down" part that can happen without us realising it. It can occur slowly over a long period of time, or it can be a rapid process, for some people showing up within an hour or so.

When I first learned the food I prepared for our daughter made her sick, I did what most parents do—I beat myself up with a huge dose of parent guilt. Then I got angry. I would tell everyone I spoke to about what was in the food they were eating. I didn't think about how people would feel about receiving this information until one day a good friend told me I sounded like a nut job! She told me to harness my anger and turn it into a passion which I could use to help others.

With that piece of friendly advice, I realised I could use our family's personal experience and what I'd learned in my studies to give me the courage to use my voice. With confidence and compassion, I started sharing what I learned and continue to learn, in the hope it would help other people experiencing the same challenges I faced.

The Mad Food Science Program

Once my husband recovered from his depression, and our family was well on the path of eating healthy real food, I began building my own health coaching practice, called "The Root Cause". I wanted to help other adults who were suffering from depression or burnout and show them how food and lifestyle could make their lives better - getting back to the heart of what was truly important (hence the name).

Around this time our daughter started getting teased about the contents of her healthy lunchbox food, to the point she would return home shaking from not eating all day out of embarrassment or fear of being teased. I spoke with the class teacher, who thought our daughter's lunches were amazing. I was invited to run a short workshop on a Friday afternoon to teach my daughter's class all about healthy food, in an attempt to stop the bullying. I called it "The Mad Food Science Program", and all weekend I got swamped with messages from parents, amazed at their child's new approach to food. I was invited to teach the rest of the school, then neighbouring schools.

In the back of my mind I'd joined the dots between the workshop I ran with our daughter's school, and the children's health statistics in Australia. Israel and I also talked about the next phase of our lives as a family, and we'd decided we'd like to travel the country rather than get into enormous levels of debt to buy a home in Sydney.

Over dinner and a few glasses of wine on our wedding anniversary, I shared my plan: create a big mobile billboard out of a bus, travel Australia, and do mobile health coaching and workshops while we travelled. With some more brainstorming, our Australian Tour to Transform Children's Health was born.

The Australian Tour to Transform Children's Health

For over two years, as a family, we travelled one and a half laps of Australia in our big green bus, visiting over ninety schools and reaching over 20,000 children, parents and teachers with our Mad Food Science Program. We learned more on our tour than you could ever learn from reading books or watching the news or reading the newspaper. We were on the ground, at the grass roots with parents, children and teachers, and it was eye opening. We gained a deep understanding of what is happening for parents and their children in relation to food choices, in a great variety of schools, across various regions and demographics. We also gained an understanding from talking to teachers about how food was impacting schools.

Here's a snippet of what we learnt.
- **Processed lunchbox food has become normal**. Many Australian Children are eating 2-4 packet foods in their lunchbox every day;
- **A great majority of parents are stressed and time poor.** This is consistent right around Australia. Parents are packing lunchboxes for convenience, without understanding the

impact the convenience food may have on their children's health, learning or the environment;

- **Kids just want to fit in.** Everyone wants processed packet food because their friends are eating it. If a child doesn't have packet food, they feel "not normal". They are often told this by their friends or that their lunch looks disgusting. This was my daughter's experience in year 2 at school; she felt "not normal" because the healthy food I packed in her lunchbox led to her classmates teasing her.
- **Teachers are spending vast amounts of time managing behaviour rather than educating.** The combination of managing children's behaviour and the requirements of a very full curriculum is creating unnecessary and undue stress for teachers.
- **Many parents say their kids are fussy eaters.** This is making meal times more stressful. Parents are buying more packets of processed food because that is what they believe and perceive their kids will eat at school. They don't want their children to go hungry.
- **Lunchbox foods are creating an enormous amount of waste.** In one school study of 320 students, they collected two washing baskets of single use plastic, per day, just from lunchboxes. When projected out across for a year, the school realised a small shipping container could be filled with the waste from children's lunchboxes alone. Other schools who have been seriously looking at sustainability have discovered similar results.

The foods being packed in lunchboxes are affecting children's long-term health, their behaviour, concentration, teacher stress, and creating a huge amount of environmental waste. The convenience is costing us in so many ways.

Kids Will Eat Real Food

Towards the end of our Australian Tour in 2017, in conjunction with forward thinking Principal Susan Hilliar, we tested the theory that in a peer environment, children will happily eat fruits and vegetables.

The Real Food Lunchbox Project involved feeding a school of 320 children real food of fruits, vegetables, dips and smoothies for recess and lunch. We asked parents to send a main lunch, and no packet food. For eight weeks, children ate real foods, fully-funded by a crowdfunding campaign we ran with our amazing community. The study included even those whose parents who thought their children wouldn't eat the fruits and vegetables and so would starve.

The outcome was significant. The children ate the fruit and vegetables served because their friends were eating it. The children started to feel healthier. They slept better. They had more energy. Their teachers saw a difference in classroom behaviour and performance too. Parents noticed a difference at home with children's sleeping, moods and attitudes towards fruits and vegetables all improving.[1]

Children just want to fit in. What they are eating doesn't matter as long as their friends are eating it!

This project gave me more determination to shine a light on what children are eating at school. I believe if we focus on improving food at school, we could improve not just the health of the children, but teacher stress levels, children's behaviour, learning and over a sustained period, academic results. And there would be a wonderful impact of reducing the amount of waste too

Putting Lunchboxes Under the Spotlight

In 2018, I was given the fantastic opportunity to share what I'd learned at the grassroots level with the Australian Federal Parliament as part of the Senate Select Committee into the Obesity Epidemic in Australia. I shared our belief that if we address what children are eating at school, we can not only improve children's health but academic results too. I shared how parents around the country have told us they are stressed and tired. Their job of getting kids to eat healthier foods is made more difficult by the food science and marketing of all the packaged and processed foods.

You can imagine my excitement when Senator Lisa Singh, Deputy Chair for the Senate Committee, mentioned our work and the Real Food Lunchbox Project in Federal Parliament in December 2018.[2]

The state of children's lunchboxes was raised as an issue in Parliament! #winning

---

Oh, but the wheels of parliament work slowly. To enact change, politicians need a majority of political parties on side, and the various industry bodies (who have deep pockets), are noisy and hold a lot of power). Fast forward sixteen months from this Committee and I have been involved in one of many community forums around the country, looking for ideas to be incorporated into a National Obesity Strategy. There are so many great ideas that have been put forward which is fantastic. However, at the Forum, it was advised that COAG (Council of Australian Governments) is only able to commit to "considering" a National Obesity Strategy by the end of 2020. That's over two years since the original Senate Select Committee Hearing.

Waiting for government to take action takes a long time because of the process. **As parents, we have the power to make changes now.**

The knowledge we gained on our Australian Tour led to us creating a vision so much larger than we ever dared before. We've seen the reality of children's health in Australia, and we're determined to do something about it. The Root Cause has now built a dedicated team of Certified Instructors around Australia trained to deliver our programs in their local communities and schools. Together with our passionate Certified Instructors, we have decided as parents, we'd like to keep lunchboxes under the spotlight.

Chapter 2
Children's Health in Australia

To fully appreciate the background of how lunchbox foods are impacting your child's learning, behaviour and health, it's important to get a reality check on children's health in Australia.

Australia is amid a children's health crisis and unless action is taken and taken right **NOW**, the health of our children will continue to decline.

Please don't get me wrong. Australia is one of the luckiest countries on the planet, and we have so much to be grateful for. While current climate conditions prove to be challenging, compared to many countries, we have better access to fresh food and water. We have an excellent health care system, and we are not in the grip of any wars or conflicts. I'm not making this statement to be dramatic or alarmist, or to incite fear and despair. However, there are many research studies showing that despite our abundance, wealth, and health care, our children's health statistics are worsening.

Let's have a quick look at the vital statistics for Australian children.

- 24.9% of our children aged 5-17 are now overweight or obese[3]
- A whopping 46% of young adults aged 18-24 are now overweight or obese. This does not start at this age; it creeps in over years of consuming poor quality foods and lack of exercise[4]
- 7.4% of our children aged 4-17 now have ADHD[5]
- 6.9% of our children aged 4-17 now have an anxiety disorder[6]
- 2.8% of our children aged 4-17 now have a depressive disorder[7]
- 10-16% of students are perceived by their teachers to have learning difficulties[8]
- 1 in 63 children are estimated to have autism[9]
- Australia has one of the highest asthma rates in the world[10]
- Children as young as 10 are being diagnosed with type 2 diabetes. Once referred to adult onset diabetes, this was not initially considered a childhood disease but has now become one[11]
- Australia has one of the highest rates of food allergies in children, in the world[12]
- 94% of children do not eat enough fruits and vegetables[13]
- Children 4-8 years old are on average eating 4.8 serves of discretionary foods per day[14]
- Children 9-13 years old are on average eating 6.2 serves of discretionary foods per day[15]
- 58% of the family's weekly food budget is now being spent on discretionary foods[16].

There's no doubt these statistics are alarming and are the reason for my statement earlier about Australia being amid a children's health crisis. By any objective viewpoint, our kids are eating too much of the wrong thing, experiencing more and more chronic and lifestyle illnesses, and getting sicker year after year.

The Many Factors at Play

This crisis has been unfolding and gaining strength for more than a decade. The human species, physiologically speaking, has not changed dramatically but the environment in which we live has changed radically. The modern lifestyle has a massive role to play in the current growing health crisis. Physical activity has declined and the way we eat has changed dramatically. The volume of toxins we are exposed to daily has increased exponentially. The amount of time spent on screens has increased too.

Parents right around the country have shared with us how stressed and time poor they are just trying to make ends meet. We need weekends for downtime. Technology use is higher in children on weekends, indicating it is used as a method of downtime for children[17]. When it comes to food, convenience through packets, jars, pouches and sachets come to the rescue.

Our food supply has been changing for the last thirty or more years. Many local fruit and vegetable shops (green grocers) have closed. Our three major supermarkets (Coles, Woolworths and Aldi) now dominate, predict and determine household spending. Astonishingly, recent studies show Australians are now spending over half of their weekly food budget on discretionary food—foods which are not part of the five food groups we need for health[18].

Discretionary foods are meant to be **sometimes or occasional** foods. Yet most Australian families are eating them daily. Many Australian children are having at least two of these discretionary foods in their lunchbox every day. To be clear, most of these discretionary foods used to be called "junk foods" or "treat foods" because years ago, parents recognised they shouldn't be eaten every day. Our bodies do not need these foods, and it's questionable whether our body knows how to use them. However, if you watch TV, listen to the radio, and scour the supermarket catalogues, you could be excused for thinking these packets are perfect for lunchboxes and for everyday eating.

Over the last decade or more, there has been considerable focus on health in relation to the role of physical activity and certain elements of food such as fat and sugar. Doctors and Personal Trainers will tell you that 80% of our health comes from what we eat. In fact, Dr Charlotte Middleton, Integrative GP, shares this statement:

"You cannot out-exercise a poor diet."

It's Not Just About How We Look

A common misconception is that being overweight or obese is all about what we can see on the outside. However, studies reveal it doesn't matter what we look like on the outside. It is what's happening on the inside of our bodies that matters. The studies identified a condition called Metabolically Obese, Normal Weight (MONW) or also called Skinny Fat or Thin on the Outside, Fat on the Inside (TOFI). This is where on the outside, people look healthy, yet on the inside fat is being stored around their internal organs.

To the best of my research, there are no studies on this for Australian children, but a study on American teens revealed 37% of so-called skinny kids had at least one sign of pre-diabetes[19]. These signs include high blood pressure, high blood sugar or high cholesterol. Given the adult history of Australians closely following the American diet and lifestyle habits, it is highly possible and probable Australian children are likely to be on a similar health path as the American children.

This is another reason this fabulous country, Australia, needs a strong focus on what we eat! We need to be asking and answering the questions: "What's In My Food?" and "What is this food potentially doing to my health and the health of my family?"

The elephant in the room is the packaged foods which have become normal in our children's lunchboxes. These foods are supposed to be "sometimes or occasional foods" (and in small amounts) yet are being eaten every day. The daily over-consumption of these foods is contributing to the decline in children's health. We need to increase the amount of fruit and vegetables kids eat and reduce the amount of processed packet food they are eating.

The Root Cause believes investing in improving school lunchboxes and food at school is a prevention strategy for Australia's Childhood Health crisis. Our waning academic results will benefit too.

School is the one place where most Australian children will be forty weeks out of the year. We know kids just want to fit in. We believe if we focus on getting more children eating fruits and vegetables at school and reducing processed food, the more normal it will become for kids to eat fruits and vegetables. And the more likely this behaviour will carry over to home too.

The Importance of School Lunchbox Food

Between 30-40 % of what your child eats Monday to Friday comes from the food in their lunchbox (or from what they order at the school canteen). Food children eat at school needs to support their growth, development and learning.

A considerable amount of the processed, packaged foods being included in lunchboxes contains little nutrition and the energy provided is short lived. Packaged foods are putting children are on an energy roller coaster. They eat and gain a burst of energy, then their energy levels crash. Unfortunately, the crash happens in the classroom.

Some ingredients, specifically the additives and preservatives in these foods, have been identified as potentially contributing to behaviour problems, learning difficulties, hyperactivity, asthma, sleep disturbance, headaches, allergies, eczema and more. It is true, not all children will be affected. You don't know if your child is being affected until you try not eating foods with these additives and preservatives for a period of time. Francine Bell, from Additive Free Kids, advises some parents see the difference in their children in as little as a week after removing certain additives and preservatives from their food. It is questionable whether our bodies know how to process ingredients that are synthetically made or derived from a natural source before being processed in a laboratory.

"A number of artificial substances and colours and sweeteners are created synthetically. And some of the substances they're derived from, I have concerns about whether they even belong in the human body."

DR LIBBY WEAVER,
FROM FMTV DOCU-SERIES TRANSCENDENCE.

Whilst on our Australian Tour, it surprised us to discover most schools allocate just 10-15 minutes for eating lunch. The preliminary research by the school before The Real Food Lunchbox Project indicated at school, when eating, children prioritise eating their processed, packaged food first. If they still have time to eat, they will start on their main lunch or their fruit.

This is consistent with discussions I've had with school groundskeepers who tell stories of bins being loaded with half-eaten sandwiches and pieces of fruit with bites out of them. The ABC's War On Waste Program also identified this phenomenon at Kiama High School where students completed an analysis on the composition of their bins. They found loads of empty packets and bottles, and many partially eaten sandwiches.

As a parent, this is something to be aware of. When you send your child to school with packet foods, a main lunch and perhaps a piece of fruit, it is likely your child will eat the packaged food first and may or may not eat the real food you have packed. If we want our children to eat more food that will help them grow, develop and learn, we need to minimise the amount of processed food, so they focus on eating the real food their bodies need, and have plenty of time to eat it during their breaks.

Lunchboxes are important, and they don't have to be difficult. Pack more fruits and vegetables and reduce the packaged food.

Common Parent Responses

As we travelled Australia and from our social media pages, we often and repeatedly hear common comments from parents and grandparents. You may think some of these yourself, or perhaps you've had people say these things to you. Please remember, there is no judgement. As you begin this journey into discovering the truth behind the food our children are eating, wherever you are at is perfect. This is your journey as a parent, and you need to do what you feel is right for your family. Here are the most common types of reactions or responses we've received:

1. "I had no idea their food could affect them like that!"

We discovered there were many parents who did not know, nor understand, the connection between food and how it makes us feel. When parents learned the significance of the ingredients in much of the food they were feeding their children, it shocked them. They had no idea what was in most of the foods they were feeding their family. Parents assume the food must be okay because it's allowed to be sold on the supermarket shelf. These same parents accepted they needed to make a change for the health of their children. We have many testimonials from parents who now make feeding their children real food a priority.

As you read this book, if you find yourself shocked *and* ready for change, visit our website for loads of free resources and recipes to help you make a change. You may also wish to consider the programs we offer to help empower you and your children to make better food choices. Visit **www.therootcause.com.au** to find out more.

2. "I don't have time to do anything about it"

By far one of the biggest comments we get from parents who either already knew this information or learned it, is: "I don't have time." I like to reframe this and ask them to consider: "How much time do you waste arguing with your kids or trying to get your kids to sleep better?"

What if you could halve the time you spent arguing with the kids or if you could get a full night sleep because your child slept through the night? How would that feel? As the saying goes, you need to spend a little time, to make time. Spending a little time planning and preparing more real food can save you time, money and improve your family relationships.

At this point, some parents seek help and start making small slow steady changes. Others turn a blind eye to what they have learned because it's too hard to think about how it can fit into their lives. I like to think this information is always at the back of their mind and I take comfort in knowing when the time is right for them, they will take action.

If you feel like this, know you are not alone. Please use all the free resources we have on our website (**www.therootcause.com.au**) to help or to consider the programs we offer to help empower you and your children to make better food choices.

3. "How can I possibly change?"

Many parents understand the information we share, and they want to make a change, but for many, change seems an impossible challenge. Many are dealing with children who are fussy eaters, have sensory issues, have been diagnosed with ADHD/ADD or have severe allergies.

Many of these parents also tell us how their children love their white, carb-heavy foods and they couldn't possibly see how they could get their kids to eat fruits and vegetables. While these scenarios might seem difficult, time is the key. The white carb foods are often part of the problem. Kids gravitate to them and unfortunately they are the foods that impact a child's gut health. When a child's gut health is compromised, many exhibit the different symptoms and behaviour patterns they struggle with and cause so much tension at home. Fussy eating, ADD & ADHD, eczema, allergies, disturbed sleep patterns, loud and boisterous, maybe even destructive behaviour.

If you feel like this, then you are not alone. Please know there are many practitioners out there who can help you. Seek the support of a nutritionist, naturopath, integrative GP or a feeding specialist. I have listed some I know and trust in the back of the appendix of this book.

4. "I don't believe you."
Life would be boring if we were all the same. Some parents, even after learning what's in the food they are feeding their children, still hold the belief if it's on the supermarket shelf, it's okay. To some extent, there was denial anything could be wrong with the food or children's health.

Some of the most common comments we received were:
* I ate that when I was growing up and I am okay
* Let kids be kids
* Stop being the fun police
* A little bit won't hurt anyone
* Stop trying to food shame people
* My kids aren't affected by the foods they eat
* Everything in moderation.

In response to this, I would say something like, "Even the biscuits and the lollies you ate when you were growing up are likely to have different ingredients today". Or "For many of us parents, this food wasn't part of our everyday food and so it was a little sometimes. Now it's no longer a little, and sometimes, it's every day—breakfast, lunch, snacks and dinner." Our kids are eating processed foods every day. The only way we will ever know if they are being affected by it, is to remove it and see what, if any, change takes place. Processed food has infiltrated the way most Australians eat, to the point we no longer recognise it as processed food. It is so normal, so naturally we don't see it for what it is: "processed".

At first, I found it tough dealing with this denial because we so desperately want to help the children of Australia be the best healthiest version of themselves they can be. There is sufficient research showing for a majority of children, what children learn to eat at home, will become what they eat when they leave home. I so desperately wanted to change what children were eating at home, so when they leave home, they would always return to eating real food, even if for a while they chose junk food. I realise; however, our job is to raise awareness by sharing information. It's a parent's job to work out how best to use this information. To do something with it or to ignore it.

Food is Highly Emotive

Being brutally honest here, food is a highly emotive topic. Every parent has the right to feed their children the way they wish. This book is not about telling you how to feed your child, it's about raising your awareness of what is happening in Australia to our children. It's about understanding the food we're sending our kids to school with, daily, may impact them physically, emotionally, behaviourally, intellectually and socially. It's about how this food is not just affecting them, but the world they are growing up in too.

Before every school term starts, the marketing campaigns for lunchbox foods announce their brilliance, convenience and suitability.

Some slogans and activities you may see are:
- "Lunchbox Friendly"
- "Perfect for Lunchboxes"
- "Lunchbox Ready"
- "Freeze for Lunchboxes"

- "Making School Easy"
- Food brands aligning themselves with specific lunchboxes
- Bonus offers. E.g. A set of name labels, vouchers for stores that sell stationery
- Exclusive product ranges only available at specific supermarket/ stores

When it's back to school time, there are yellow sale dockets throughout the supermarkets aisles selling foods dressed up to be lunchbox friendly. Companies pay supermarkets substantially to have displays of their products and their sales at various vantage points throughout the supermarket. The yellow "special" tags are just one of the various tactics designed to drive purchasing behaviour. This is generally known as trolleyology.[20] Such tactics have a way of blurring consumers' vision, understanding and perception of what food is the best for our school lunchboxes.

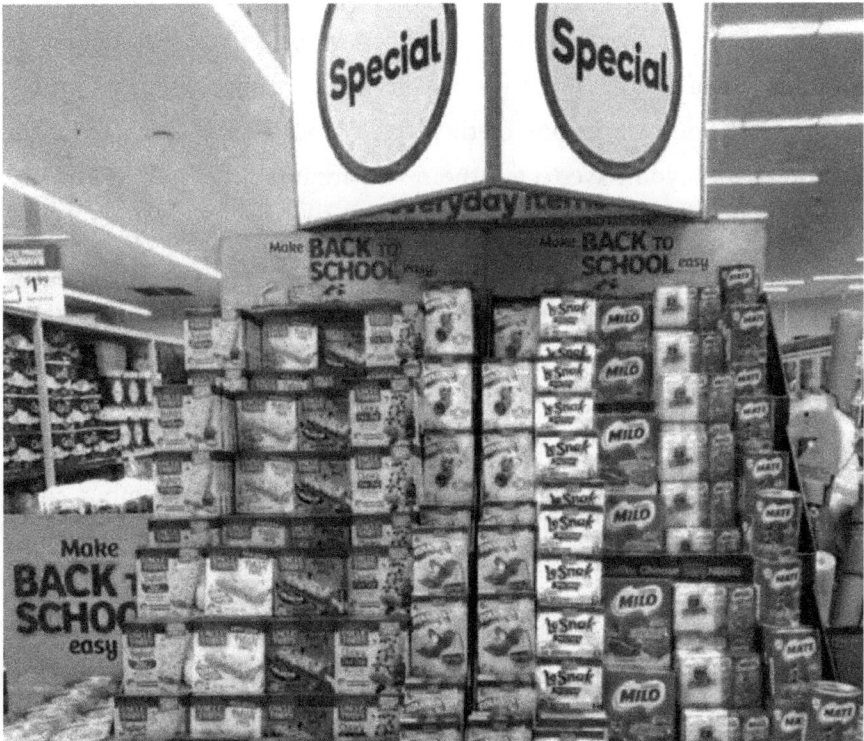

The media are great at publishing stories and articles on what to pack in school lunchboxes. They are also good at hyping up stories about the school who dares to send notes home to parents about what to pack in school lunchboxes. This commonly spikes the fury and indignation of parents. Common responses include – "How dare they tell me what to pack?", "It's none of their business!", "They're not trained in nutrition." and so on.

It is time to address this because the food in children's lunchboxes can affect their ability to behave in class, to socialise in the playground, to work amicably with the other students and be respectful to the teachers. As parents sending our children to school, we are outsourcing every aspect of their growth and development, socialisation and learning to the school for the day. What the children are eating at school is very much the school's business. Teachers are on the receiving end of the effects of what's in children's lunchboxes every day.

Let's think about this a little differently. Let's say you work in an office, and every single day you keep getting calls that belong to another department. The calls are generally from upset customers. Every time you receive one of these calls, you receive abuse from the customer then you have to tell them you are unable to help them. The customer becomes even more annoyed with the next person when you transfer them. This problem is really affecting how you feel about coming to work. What would you do? Would you just put up with it every day? Or would you talk to your manager and ask for the IVR on the phone to be made clearer, so people were directed to the right department and you didn't have to deal with those calls anymore? In most businesses, if a problem like this existed, a staff member could ask for it to be fixed and they could improve the process for everyone's benefit.

I personally believe it is appropriate and relevant for schools to ask parents to send children to school with food which contributes to calmer, happier children. Children who are better able to learn from both positive and negative experiences, to socialise, play and interact with other children and adults. Isn't this why we send our children to school? Addressing what's in our children's lunchboxes isn't about lunchbox shaming on the part of school. It is a healthy approach for schools to take. Healthy for the children's bodies and minds; for the teachers; for the learning environment, the social environment and as equally importantly to planet Earth's health too.

One aim I have for you from reading this book is for you to recognise–and ignore–marketing hype. Then you can pack lunchbox foods, including packets if you wish, from a position of power. Then you can consciously choose foods that work for your family and give your children the best possible chance for long-term health and learning.

A Simple Way to Talk to Your Children

To help you on your way, we have a few messages we use in our Mad Food Science Program to empower children that you can learn for yourself, and talk with your children about:

We have One Body for Life, so we need to fuel it every day with foods our body needs and knows how to use.
- Eat more fruits and vegetables.
- Minimise your processed, packaged foods (e.g. if you have two packets today, tomorrow just have one).
- If you want to have processed, packaged food, **ask: "What's In My Food?"**
- The best drink for school is water (keep juice and flavoured milks for home).
- Eating more fruits and vegetables and less processed food is good for your One Body For Life, and good for our One Planet For Life.

Chapter 3
Lunchboxes: Then and Now

Before we explore some of the issues surrounding today's lunchbox foods, it's important to understand where we've come from. I was fortunate to meet Susan Hilliar, Principal of two schools and a teacher since 1985, on our Australian Tour, and I invited her to write this next section. Susan drew on over thirty years of teaching, to bring us this insight into what has changed in her experience during that time.

The Change in the Lunchbox Over Thirty Years – Susan Hilliar

When I began teaching in 1985, the lunchbox contents looked very different to today's lunchboxes. Most children ate fresh fruit whilst playing and most children had a sandwich and a homemade piece of cake or a biscuit. We rarely saw packaged food from tubs, packets of chips, plastic cheese products or a bottle of juice. Children slurped water from school bubblers and shared their orange segments with one another while playing. The staple fast food for a hungry child was bananas.

Fast forward to today's lunchbox, and we see very different contents which I am unable to say is nutritious food to service a child for a six-hour learning day.

The contents of these lunchboxes no longer discriminate between the socially disadvantaged or the affluent. They no longer show which children come from single parent families or families where parents are working or not. The lunchbox is now an indication of the time poor parent who will move through the supermarket aisles tossing in packet after packet of lunchbox contents because it's what all children have packed for school. Those few children who do have a nutritious lunchbox are seen as "slightly different" or "healthy" or have one of "those parents" who is a vegetarian or vegan.

Our new generation of teachers do not have the hindsight to know how the lunchbox has changed over the years. These teachers have not seen the change to children's concentration over the last three and half decades. Nor attitudes change of tired parents giving into the pesky child nagging at the supermarket trolley to include those snacks everyone eats at school.

As Principal of two schools, I have seen firsthand the difficulty of trying to raise awareness of the changed contents of the lunchboxes. When an inquiry is opened up about the lunchbox contents, the response was almost always the same—an offended parent defending the time poor family. They say the lunchbox was better consumed at school with preservative enhanced pre-packaged food rather than a child coming home having not touched the homemade fruit and veg based lunchbox.

To carve a new way of thinking, a new way of developing a peer supported approach to whole school fruit and vegetable lunchbox required a different model of delivery. An eight-week trial of the whole school "Real Food Lunchbox Project" demonstrated when all children eat fresh fruit and vegetables together at school, then they all do it. Once families were asked to commit beyond the lunchbox provided trial, sadly, the contents of the lunchbox resumed back to their pre-packaged preservative snacks. Concentration and behaviour returned to where they were before the trialled lunchbox project. The evidence collected throughout the trial period undoubtedly showed an increase in concentration, calmer students, with a reduction in children in trouble throughout the school day.

When children were taught to read the contents of their own lunchbox snacks, their biggest challenge came in trying to educate their parents while out shopping. Parents didn't have time to debate with their children. Shopping was an in and out experience and one to be done as quickly as possible.

Our lunchbox contents have become the window into family life. It appears our education system has not yet made the link between the contents of school lunches with that of learning outcomes. My greatest hope is there is a willingness from those in government to take on a whole school lunchbox project. They'll discover the evidence we found behind the data that supports a fruit and vegetable snack based lunchbox has profound results for children, their learning, their behaviour and their health.

A Look Inside Today's Common Lunchbox

Having read Susan's perspective on lunchboxes over the last thirty years, now let's take a deep dive into what's in common lunchboxes today. To help, I've included a few photos to give us a visual look at some of the most common lunches we've come across. These are actual lunchboxes from The Real Food Lunchbox Project undertaken at a NSW School of 320 students. This project found on average students were having between two and four packets in their lunchbox a day.

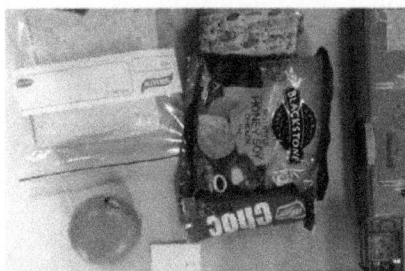

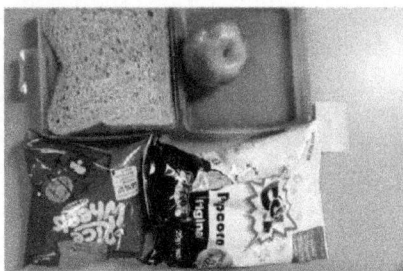

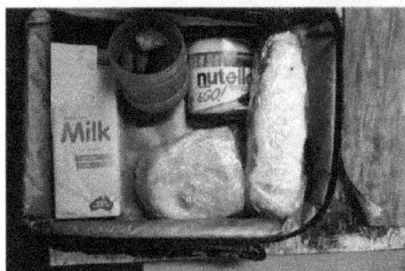

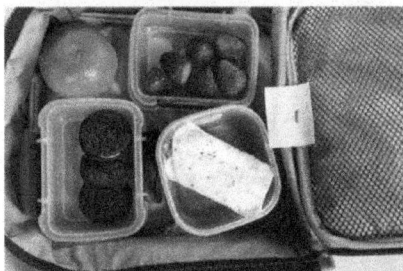

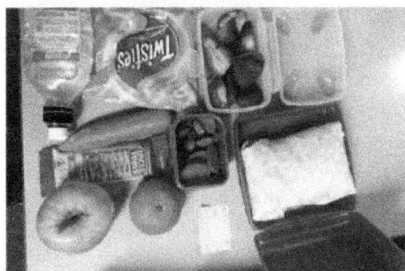

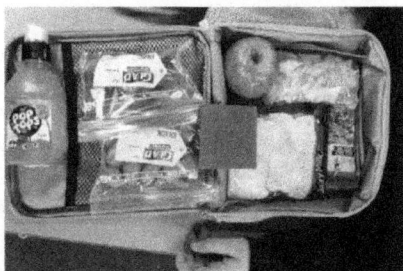

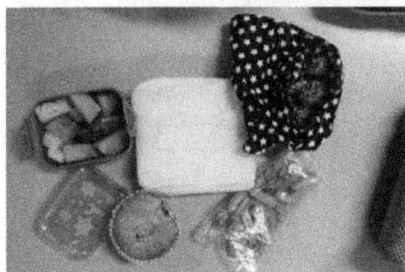

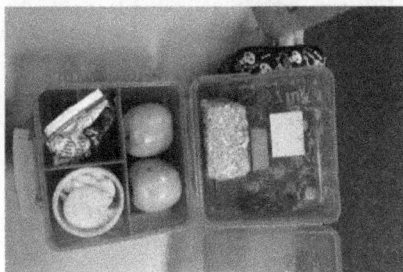

From what we witnessed firsthand travelling Australia, and from what teachers have told us, these lunchboxes are pretty representative of lunchboxes around Australia.

The Real Food Lunchbox Project also identified that students generally gravitated to their packaged food first, and if there was time left to eat their lunch, then they would move onto their sandwich / main lunch or their fruit.

As we travelled Australia, and even today, teachers tell us about the impacts these foods are having on children in the classroom. Here's just a few examples of what we hear.

Karen ____ I see it all the time - rubbish in lunch boxes and then half an hour later they want to put their head on the desk!

Like · Reply · Message · 44w   👍 1

Sue-Ellen ____ Over my career as a primary school teacher i have seen the changes to the students recess and lunch! It is absolutely horrifying!! I am sickened by the amount of processed, junk (can't even be called food!) children are being given (by adults) to consume every day! Students health, well being and learning are all hugely impacted. I strongly feel it is a form of child abuse!

Like · Reply · Message · 1d   👍 3

Pauline ____ I've taught at schools who do have strict lunchbox rules and not only is their behaviour better but not one of them are overweight. In comparison with schools where kids are eating all sort of junk (plus it being served in the tuckshop) kids are hungry, tired, have increased behaviour issues and weight problems. I stand with you 😊

Like · Reply · Message · 2w   👍 4

The Science of How Food Impacts Children

There is plenty of scientific studies that support what teachers have told us. Dietitian Madison Hille reviewed studies for this book, and I share some of the most pertinent findings that support what teachers are telling us:

- Children behave significantly better in class and remain more "on task" in the afternoon after a nutritious lunch.[21]
- Poor nutritional quality is independently associated with symptoms of attention-deficit hyperactivity disorder.[22]
- Nutrition, particularly in the short-term, is believed to impact upon individual behaviour, (e.g. concentration, activity levels). These behaviours have the potential to affect school performance and interaction with peers, and to compromise self-esteem[23].
- The research shows that having a healthy, balanced diet improves brain capacity, maximizes cognitive capabilities, and improves academic performance in school-age children. Alternatively, the research also shows that having too much junk food and an unhealthy diet decreases academic performance by limiting the amount of information to the brain.[24]

In addition to the above studies, there was a 4 year study of over 1,000,000 students across 803 schools in New York City Public Schools. The study took place in 1979 to 1983. The study involved changing the school lunches, so they had reduced sugar and additives that affected learning and behaviour. The results were astounding[25]:

- 75,000 students were no longer considered to be learning disabled
- The schools' national ranking went from 11% below average to 5% above average
- "No other school district reported such a large gain above the rest of the nation so quickly" -

Today's Lunchbox Data Analysis

Right around the country, teachers and principals have told they feel their hands are tied in talking to parents about lunchboxes. As such, in 2019, The Root Cause started offering schools the chance to participate in a Food and Waste Survey when they participated in The Mad Food Science Program. The outcome is schools receive a Food and Waste Benchmark Report providing them with specific data about their school. This gives them concrete and meaningful data to be having conversations with the parenting community.

From data we collected on almost 6,000 lunchboxes from 35 schools, across 343 classes, this is what a common lunchbox looks like statistically speaking[26]:

- 88% of students bring lunches from home
- 2% had no lunch
- The balance bought some or all of their lunch from the canteen
- 2 packet foods per lunchbox
- 1 fruit per lunchbox
- 0.4 vegetables per lunchbox
- 70% contain a sandwich
- 73% of sandwiches were white bread
- 50% of the sandwiches contained a spread such as vegemite, honey, jam

Our National Data Partner, Sync or Swim, have generously donated their time for the greater good of this book. They have taken the data collected from the schools surveyed, and the data for the more than 480 common lunchbox foods we've listed in this book and completed additional analysis. This has allowed us to have a look at the composition of just the lunchbox packet foods (not the rest of the lunchbox) from those surveyed.

What we can tell you is that, looking specifically at just the packet foods, the average lunchbox contains:

- 29 ingredients
- 3.6 teaspoons of sugar (This is alarming. In terms of the World Health Organisations recommendations, this is about what they should have across the **entire** day)

- 148mg sodium
- 9 additives, 4 of which can be potentially linked to hyperactivity, learning difficulty and behavioural issues.
- 20% of packet foods are chips, 17% are muesli and other sorts of bars, 15% are savoury crackers, 15% are sweet biscuits, 10% are chocolate and lollies, 10% are juices and flavoured milks, 8% are yoghurts and other pouches, the balance is fruit or jelly cups and the like.

The purpose of sharing the data with you is to show how this backs up the visual data. This data also supports the anecdotal evidence we gathered as we travelled Australia. Processed packaged food now dominates school lunchboxes.

I acknowledge there are other factors than just food that can affect children's behaviour, like technology usage and lack of sleep. However, food has become the elephant in the room. It's emotive nature means it rarely gets tackled. In sharing this information, I am bringing up the elephant in the room, front and centre. I hope you see what a problem packaged food has become in our lunchboxes and why we need to start talking about The Lunchbox Effect.

Fuelling Our Bodies

The fuel we run on as humans is, obviously, our food and drinks. But let's use a car as an analogy, to help illustrate a point.

With a car, there is a straight message in the user manual—use this specific kind of fuel (e.g. Diesel, Unleaded, Premium). If we don't use that kind of fuel, the engine will run poorly, or possibly break down. As car owners, we know what kind of fuel our vehicle requires, so we use only that kind of fuel. Similarly, animals in the wild inherently know what they need to eat and drink as their fuel, and so they eat and drink accordingly.

As humans, we have the luxury of choosing from a wide variety of fuels, although there are some that are better for our "engine" than others. The Australian Dietary Guidelines provide a recommendation of what foods and drinks we should eat to maintain a healthy body and mind. They categorised this into five basic food groups[27].

- Vegetables and legumes/beans
- Fruit
- Grain (cereal) foods, mostly wholegrain and/or high cereal fibre varieties
- Lean meats and poultry, fish, eggs, tofu, nuts and seeds and legumes/beans
- Milk, yoghurt cheese and/or alternatives, mostly reduced fat

Discretionary foods, which includes most processed, packaged foods, do not feature in these 5 food groups. They are listed down the bottom with these words "Only sometimes and in small amounts." Yet, discretionary foods dominate shelf space at the supermarket, and make up a significant portion of the average child's lunchbox.

A Note on the Australian Dietary Guidelines

It is my personal belief and that of many nutritionists and naturopaths I have spoken to, that these dietary guidelines need updating. The categorisation of mostly reduced fat for dairy is a carry-over from years gone by where fat was demonised. Most low fat foods have been bolstered with added sugar or additives to add back in the taste that has been lost by removing the fat. Many of these low fat, but subsequently high sugar items are allowed on canteen menus.

When expressing my concern to a government health promotion officer about the amount of sugar in these foods and drinks, I was advised they are "a vehicle for getting calcium into children". Don't you think it's odd that the canteen guidelines are trying to fix the problem of getting children to have calcium? However, by feeding them up on foods and drinks made with flavours created in a chemistry lab, they're loading them up with sugar.

The simple fact is the food and drinks we have are our body's fuel sources. It stands to reason the amount and quality of the food and drinks we consume will have a bearing on our performance.

The best foods for our children's lunchboxes are those which will help them thrive. You'll learn more about these foods in the next chapter.

Chapter 4
The Food Kids Need to Thrive

A Simple Way to Talk to Your Children

I will break this down in the simple terms we share with children in The Mad Food Science Program because I want you to be able to explain this to your children. Then I will introduce Jo Atkinson, Nutritionist, to share a deeper explanation of how the food we eat is incredibly important to how well our body works and that nutrients are essential to our cells to function properly. When our cells aren't functioning properly, our body isn't functioning properly. This is important information that we adults can all benefit from understanding.

In the Mad Food Science Program our Certified Instructors talk to the children about their body and the fuel it needs to make them go and be the best version of themselves they can be. You can use these messages to have conversations with your own kids:

In the same way a car needs the right fuel to run smoothly, so too does your body. You need to put the right fuel into your body so you can run smoothly. With a car, you have a manual, and it tells you the kind of fuel your car needs. Your car has gauges that tell you when to add oil and water. But unlike a car, you have the choice of fuel (food and drinks) you put in your body. You don't have gauges on your body, so it's super important for you to tune in and listen to your body.

The next important message you can share is this. When a car gets to ten or twelve-years-old, it's likely to cost extra money for repairs. For adults, we can trade the car in and get another car, usually a younger one. You can't do this with your body. You only have your One Body For Life. This means every day you need to fuel your body with foods that help your body, and only sometimes have fuel (foods and drinks) that don't help your body. Every day is straight forward: Sunday, Monday, Tuesday, Wednesday, Thursday, Friday, Saturday.

In The Mad Food Science Program we ask children to share what *sometimes* mean. They know and say it means:

- Not every day
- Once in a blue moon
- Special occasions
- Once a week
- Once a month
- Two or three times a week

Now, you might like to ask your children to tell you what *sometimes* means.

Did you notice children know *sometimes* is not every day? Yet, many children, every day are unconsciously eating sometimes foods in their lunchbox. This is because sometimes foods **have been normalised in school lunchboxes.**

We do only have one body for life. Every day we need to choose fuel–food and drinks–which help our body, and only sometimes have fuel which doesn't help our body.

We encourage you to have these conversations at home, so your children understand why the food and drink they have is so important for their body.

A Deeper Chat for Adults

Jo Atkinson, Nutritionist shares her incredible, professional knowledge on the body, its function and its nutrient requirements.

Eleven different systems make up our bodies. Every system in the body requires essential nutrients that most people are familiar with proteins, fats, carbohydrates, vitamins, minerals and water. You may think of these as foods, and they are. Food provides energy and the raw materials every cell in our body needs to function.

You know the saying "You are what you eat"? Well, we are!!

The foods we eat get broken down into their smallest parts and absorbed by our body. Then they're sent to cells and tissues to build, repair and maintain them - making these foods a part of us.

If we are what we eat, that makes the food we eat incredibly important to how well our body works. These nutrients are essential because our cells need them to function properly. When our cells aren't functioning properly, our body isn't functioning properly.

When those nutrients aren't available, the body systems break down or malfunction. When this happens, we experience negative signs and symptoms and we reduce the body's ability to fight off disease.

We also have the additional challenge of our supermarket aisles being full of products that whilst labelled as "food", contain ingredients our bodies have not evolved to deal with and contain very little, if any, of the nutrition we need. These ingredients, we know them as colours, flavours and preservatives, can damage our body and cause poor health.

So, our children's growing health problems can often be tied back to not having enough of the right nutrients. Or eating foods that lack nutrition and introduce artificial ingredients into their bodies that cause damage.

Some signs and symptoms your child may not be getting the nutrition they need from the foods they're eating include;

- Fussy eating
- Poor sleep
- Anxiety
- Eczema
- Recurring infections (ear infections/tonsillitis)
- Behavioural or learning problems

The Connection Between the Gut and the Brain

Ever had a "gut feeling" about something? Or gotten butterflies in your tummy when you felt nervous? This is the work of your gut communicating with your brain and vice versa via the two-way superhighway known as the "gut-brain axis". This connection also has a significant impact on your child's immune system, their sleep patterns, their appetite and their moods.

The foods our children eat directly affect their gut microbiome— the 100 trillion microbes that live in their gut and are using the gut-brain axis to communicate with your child's brain. These microbes help to digest the foods they eat, produce vitamins including B12, thiamine and riboflavin and vitamin K and also produce the neurotransmitters; serotonin and dopamine that impact your child's mood and behaviour.

For example, dopamine allows us to regulate emotional responses. Serotonin maintains mood balance and impulse control. An imbalance in these neurotransmitters can make it more difficult for your child to sit still and concentrate at school. They are being asked to do something their body cannot support.

The connection between the brain and the gut not only impacts their mood and behaviour, but also their overall health.

Why Do Kids' Growing Bodies Need Fruits and Vegetables?

What are the kinds of foods we can eat to make sure our gut stays working well and can do its job, so our cells have all the nutrients they need to keep us healthy?

Well, we all know we need to eat fruit and vegetables. Did you know less than half of Australian children are eating the recommended serving of fruit per day? And only around 1% eat the minimum recommended serves of vegetables each day?

Whole fruit and vegetables (WHOLE meaning not processed into a muesli bar, not dried, and not juice), provide the body with loads of essential nutrients we need like carbohydrates, protein, vitamins, minerals and water, plus importantly, fibre.

What Nutrients Do Children's Bodies Need to Thrive?

To thrive, not just survive, all bodies, adult and children's need macronutrients (carbohydrates, protein, fats) and water.

Carbohydrates

Carbohydrates provide the body with energy in the form of glucose. It is important to choose the right carbohydrate to avoid blood sugar imbalances for your child during the day.

Carbohydrates from vegetables, fruit, whole grains, pulses, nuts and seeds are a great source of fibre, minerals and vitamins. The fibre helps kids feel fuller for longer. It slows down the absorption of sugars into the bloodstream and it is food for many of our beneficial gut bacteria.

Ensuring your kids eat the minimum recommended servings of fruit and vegetables each day and eat a wide range of nutritious whole foods (foods close to their original source) will go a long way to helping your child to thrive.

Protein

Protein is an essential nutrient we can't live without. We are literally made of proteins! Proteins play several roles in the body including digestive enzymes (to break down our foods), build muscle (including our heart). Proteins also build our cells, neurotransmitters, hormones and DNA.

The protein we eat (from animals and plants) breaks down in the gut into amino acids. Amino acids form the building blocks for all our cells and tissues, including our immune system and our organs like the heart and lungs.

Amino acids are also important for the health of the gut itself. For example, the amino acid "glutamine" is absorbed directly into the cells that line the gut wall (and make up the mucous membrane). This makes a strong barrier against bacteria, viruses or parasites that can make us sick.

Protein intake is also essential for the production of vital neurotransmitters including; dopamine, noradrenaline, histamine and glycine. One such protein is tryptophan, a precursor for serotonin which has effects on mood and memory.

Good sources of protein include eggs, grass-fed beef, lamb, chicken, fish, nuts, seeds, legumes, spinach, asparagus, broccoli and dairy.

How much protein do kids need?

- **Children aged 1-3 years require approx. 14g of protein daily.** This may look like - 1/2 a boiled egg + 1/2 cup yoghurt + 2 slices of roast meat.

- **Children aged 4-8 years require approx. 20g of protein daily.** This may look like - 1 boiled egg + 1 small handful of mixed seeds + 1/2 cup cooked chicken.

- **Boys aged 9-13 years require approx. 40g of protein per day** This may look like - 2 fried eggs + 170g Greek yoghurt + 1 palm-sized piece of steak with steamed vegetables.

- **Girls aged 9-13 years require approx. 35g of protein per day** This may look like - 1 fried egg with ½ avocado + 50g Greek yoghurt + 1 cup lentils with steamed vegetables.

Fats

We have been told for many years eating fat is bad for us, but is it? The answer is no, eating fat is not just good for us, it's essential! **But it needs to be the right kind of fat.**

Fats are part of every single cell in your child's body and they are vital for hormone production, brain function, memory and concentration. Most of your child's nervous system—the brain, spinal column and all the nerves that branch off it are also made from fats and fat-soluble vitamins (A, D, E & K). Good fats are also beneficial to the health of our gut and the microbes living in it.

If your child appears hungry all the time, check the amount of nutritious fat in their diet. Children who eat low-fat foods eat more refined carbohydrates (bread, pasta, cereal, cakes, biscuits, processed foods) which aren't as filling.

Eating too much of any one thing isn't great for us, so for a healthy body and a healthy gut, we need diversity in our diet. This means we need to eat a variety of different fats.

The different fats including saturated fats, monounsaturated fats, polyunsaturated fats (from wholefood sources), Omega-3 and

Omega-6 fatty acids all provide benefits to the body.

These benefits include;
* Blood sugar regulation
* Brain and nervous system function and development
* Nutrient absorption and immune function
* Positive mood, mental health and behaviour.

How much fat do our kids need?

We should add **good fat** to every meal. Fats make us feel full and are essential for the absorption of fat-soluble nutrients. This can be through cooking (butter, olive oil) or added - avocado, meat, cheese, nuts.

The goal is not to count fat grams, or to limit total fat but to include quality fat sources as a sensible (and tasty) part of meals.

Good sources of healthy fats include;
* Avocados
* Grass-fed meats
* Butter
* Nuts & seeds
* Oily fish (sardines, wild salmon, herring, mackerel)
* Extra-virgin (cold pressed olive and coconut oils

Water

Our bodies are made of about 70% water. Without it, we would die. Water makes up most of our blood, digestive juices and sweat, and it's found in our organs and muscle cells. Water is used to metabolise fuel, regulate body temperature and digest food. To enable our bodies to carry out all its functions in the day, water constantly moves about and is lost in the air we breathe, urine, blood loss, sweat and even tears. Children in particular need to make sure they are continually re-hydrating, and water is the main way they regulate their body temperature.

Not drinking enough water can be one of the most common reasons for constipation in kids and even just being slightly dehydrated can cause kids to lose concentration and get headaches.

In terms of gut health, water is the only drink our kids' bodies need.

Water is the best drink option for children at school.

<u>How much water do kids need?</u>

The amount of water a child needs is influenced by the amount of activity they do, the weather temperature, and their diet and health. It's always important to remind children to drink water, but as a general guide, children up to eight years of age should have a minimum of 4-5 cups of water a day. Children above eight-years-old require at least 6-8 cups of water a day.

What Micronutrients Do Our Kids Need?

Micronutrients including iron, zinc, choline, selenium, iodine, magnesium, B vitamins, and vitamins A and C play key roles in energy metabolism and neurological processes which are all essential to your child's brain development.

We find these micronutrients in real, whole foods. You may see some of these micronutrients listed as ingredients on processed, packaged food or see the words "enriched" or "fortified" on packet foods. However, it is unlikely these micronutrients will be in the form our body needs. Enriched or fortified forms of micronutrients don't come with the nutrients they needed to help our bodies utilise them properly.

Iodine

Iodine is necessary for normal growth and development of the brain and body. Iodine is necessary for the body to produce thyroid hormones, which regulate our metabolism.

Good whole food sources of iodine include;
* Seaweed (including nori)
* Dairy (particularly full fat, unsweetened Greek yoghurt)
* Eggs
* Seafood

Iron

Iron is critical to your child because it's vital to brain development and they also need iron to transport oxygen through the blood to all the cells in their body. Iron is also an essential nutrient for many beneficial gut microbes. Fatigue, lethargy, irritability, inattention, and decreased IQ is seen in iron deficient children and have also been linked to the symptoms of ADHD.

Good whole food sources of iron include;
* Red meat
* Fish
* Eggs
* Leafy green vegetables
* Beans & legumes (beans, chickpeas, peas, lentils, peanuts).
* Nuts and seeds

Folate

When we're trying to get pregnant is the time you probably hear about the importance of folate, but it's also important in everyday life.

Studies have linked low levels of folate to depression in adolescents, while they associate optimal folate levels with positive effects on mood.

Good whole food sources of folate include;
* Leafy green vegetables
* Avocado
* Broccoli
* Legumes

Vitamin B12

Vitamin B12 helps to produce neurotransmitters in your brain, which carry chemical signals throughout our entire body, affecting your mood, energy, appetite. Vitamin B12 also helps turn the foods your children eat into energy.

Good whole food sources of vitamin B12 include;
- Beef liver
- Sardines
- Lamb
- Wild caught salmon
- Grass-fed butter
- Eggs
- Cheese

Vitamin D

Vitamin D is one of the most important micronutrients for your health. It's involved in healthy immunity, brain function and strong bones and teeth.

Good whole food sources of vitamin D include;
- Oily fish
- Cod liver oil
- Eggs
- Beef liver
- Grass-fed butter

Why Do Our Bodies Need Essential Fatty Acids?

Essential fatty acids (EFA's) are a special fat the body cannot make and therefore we must get them from the foods we eat.

EFA's include;

Omega-6 fatty acids;
- Linoleic acid (LA)
- Gamma-linolenic acid (GLA) and
- Arachidonic acid (AA)

And Omega-3 fatty acids
- Alpha-linolenic acid (ALA)
- Eicosapentaenoic acid (EPA) and
- Docosahexaenoic acid (DHA).

Essential fatty acids are important for both brain development and mental health. Research shows children deficient in these essential fats are at a higher risk of developing anxiety, depression, ADHD, bipolar disorder and antisocial behaviour.

Good whole food sources of EFA's include;
- Oily fish
- Avocado
- Leafy green vegetables
- Olive oil
- Eggs
- Nuts and seeds

What Foods are Good for Brain Function?

The brain is a highly active organ which demands a high percentage of the overall daily energy requirements supplied by the food our children eat. In children between the ages of 6-12 years, 30–45% of their energy is utilised in the brain.

If children are eating foods which have little nutrition, then their brains are being starved of the nutrition they need to function properly.

The increasing number of children being diagnosed with ADHD is also a concern and one that can be directly correlated to nutritional deficiencies. Research has found a high proportion of children with ADHD are iron deficient or essential fatty acid (EFA) deficient or both. Other theories regarding nutritional disturbances associated with the development of ADHD include general under-nutrition and the increased amount of junk food that children are eating from a very young age.

One of the greatest effects of nutrition on brain functioning is on our cognition (thinking). The effects of poor diet on sleeping patterns, energy and mood all indirectly affect day to day functioning of the brain at school.

Different foods provide different nutrients which have different actions in development, maturation, growth and protection of the brain.

Foods providing nutrients that benefit the developing brains of our children include;
- Oily fish
- Berries
- Eggs
- Leafy green vegetables
- Nuts and seeds (particularly walnuts and pumpkin seeds)

Impacts of Processed Packet Lunchbox Foods on Children's Bodies and Brain

Less than 1% of Australian children are eating the minimum recommended serves of vegetables each day. One reasons for this is they eat way too much processed food which takes the place of the foods children need to eat for good health.

Highly processed and packaged foods lack the nutrients your growing child needs. Think of your kids as "under construction". They need the right raw materials to grow up strong and healthy. If they're eating more packaged foods than nutritious, whole foods, they won't have the right materials to make their growth and development happen. This can lead to health problems, both immediate and in the long term.

Nutrient deficiencies in children, particularly iron and zinc, can lead to fussy eating, impaired immune function, impaired cognitive (brain based skills) and neurological function (brain, spine and nerves). With iron deficiency, these impairments may not be reversible.

Middle childhood is also a time of rapid bone growth. Without the nutrients they need to lay down bone during this peak growth time, including calcium, vitamin D, vitamin K2, magnesium and zinc, they won't be able to reach their peak bone mass. This might stunt their growth and increase their risk of fractures and osteoporosis later in life.

Let's break down some key ingredients which turn up in processed foods that can impact your child's health.

How does added sugar affect health?

Added sugar has a massive impact on the health of our children's bodies and brains. It's in almost every processed packet lunchbox food on the market.

When your child eats a meal or snack high in sugar or refined carbohydrates, (such as muesli bars, sweetened yoghurt, or white bread) this raises their blood sugar. This causes a massive excretion of insulin from the pancreas to bring it back down again. This triggers the "flight or fight" response in the nervous system sparking off an increase of adrenalin—a ball of energy that can lead to hyperactivity, anxiety, meltdowns and disruptive behaviour.

Imagine your child has cereal for breakfast, a muesli bar for recess, and a ham and cheese sandwich for lunch with a juice box. When they get home from school, perhaps they have some flavoured crackers, chips or sweet biscuits for afternoon tea. All day they've linked their tastes and messages to the brain to sugar. Now, imagine you're trying to get them to eat their veggies at dinner time. Do you think it's likely to be an easy meal time? It's likely your child will have an aversion to veggies because it's lacking the sugar taste.

This fairly typical diet of processed foods contains a cocktail of sugar, additives, preservatives and artificial colours that set your child off on an energy rollercoaster ride with their energy going up and down all day.

Imagine a child on this rollercoaster ride, trying to sit in their chair and concentrate on what the teacher is saying to avoid getting in trouble. It's no wonder that by dinner time, when you have prepared a healthy meal for them, they won't sit still and the battle to get them to eat anything resembling "healthy" begins.

How do the fats in processed food affect health?

There are "good" kinds of fats your child's body needs for growth and development, and then there are also some types of fats that should be avoided. Good fats are usually more expensive ingredients and are therefore less likely to make their way into lunchbox packet foods.

Avoid the fats called trans fats such as "vegetable oil" and seed oils such as canola, rice bran oil and safflower oils, and they are all found in processed foods. These oils are very high in Omega-6 fatty acids and can throw out the balance of the good Omega-3 fats. Over eating Omega-6 fats can lead to inflammation which is a major cause of most chronic diseases we see now; type 2 diabetes, obesity, heart disease, IBS, asthma and cancer. These are the fats and oils that end up in lunchbox packet food.

Salt

Salt is also called sodium chloride or just sodium. Sodium is integral to health; however, you can have too much. They add salt to many processed packet foods including breakfast cereal. Many lunchbox packet foods include salt too. When eating several packet foods a day, it is easy for the salt to add up across all the packets.

Sodium doesn't have a Recommended Daily Intake (RDI). Instead, it is listed as an UL (upper limit). This is the MAXIMUM amount of sodium you should have in a day.

The daily recommended maximum amount of salt children should eat depends on age:
- Children aged 1-3 years - 2.5g daily (½ a teaspoon)
- Children aged 4-8 - 3.5g daily
- Children aged 9-13 - 5g (1 teaspoon)
- Teenagers & Adults - 5.75g

5g salt = approx. 1 teaspoon

Food labels in Australia usually give the figure for sodium rather than salt. To convert sodium to salt, multiply the sodium figure in milligrams (mg) by 2.5 and then divide by 1000 to find out how many grams of salt there is.

For example, the salt content of 200mg of sodium is:

200mg x 2.5 = 500mg of salt
500mg/1000 = 0.5g of salt

Here is a link to a handy calculator :
http://rootcau.se/saltconverter

What Advice Can I Offer You?

When I talk about the negative impact of sugar, unhealthy fats, and salt in processed foods, it can give a picture of "doom and gloom" and this is not my intention. My aim is to show you the evidence, pique your curiosity about how your child's body works and how the foods they eat impact their health, both positively and negatively.

My advice is to:

- Role model eating a wide variety of fruits and vegetables.
- Reduce the amount of processed packet foods you make available to your children.
- Increase the amount of vegetables your children are currently eating. This could be as simple as if they don't take any veggies to school normally, pack a small amount in. Start with a vegetable they like that's easy to eat.
- Include a small to moderate amount of good fats in every meal.
- Ensure your child is eating as close to the recommended amount of protein as possible.
- Make water the go-to drink in your home and in the lunchbox.

Jo Atkinson
Nutritional Medicine Practitioner BHSc (Nut Med)

PART 2

What is causing us the biggest issues now?

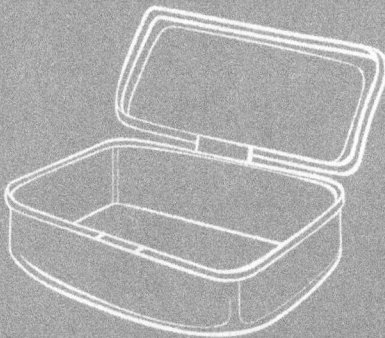

Chapter 5
The Industrialisation of Food

This topic has the potential to open a whole can of worms, so I will be clear up front. Without a doubt, in today's busy, populated world, there is a need and a place for processed, packaged food. However, at The Root Cause, we strongly believe the place for processed food comes second to eating real wholefoods.

The Blessing and Curse of Endless Variety
In food shopping we are both blessed and cursed with variety. We have so many food choices and the volume of these food choices contributes to making it difficult to make choices that are nutritious and help our bodies. There are so many claims being made on the front of packets and in marketing campaigns. Unless you stick to the perimeter of a supermarket, you will be confronted with huge

amounts of product choices, advertising, slogans and promotions—all encouraging you to buy. Even some products in the fridge section of the perimeter aisles no longer offer best choices, especially flavoured milks and flavoured yoghurts (including vanilla flavour).

It is hard to get a definitive answer to how many products there are on the supermarket shelves these days. In this book, we look at just 488 of the most common packet lunchbox foods. With such an enormous variety of options, spread across an equally enormous amount of shelf space, it's easy to see how the processed and packaged foods have become such an integral part of today's food culture.

There is a key to navigating the amount of products at the supermarket and it is to ask ONE question; "What's In My Food?" To find an answer, look at the ingredients listed on the back of the products. It is here you will discover just how many ingredients the different products each contain and how many of those ingredients you not only cannot pronounce but also how many are unrecognisable. They aren't ingredients you can purchase at the supermarket, pop in your pantry and use in your cooking. Many of the ingredients, specifically flavours, additives and preservatives are explicitly made for industrialised food processing. For example, flavour enhancer 635 also known as Disodium 5'–ribonucleotides, or preservative 282 Calcium propionate.

Common to most products are salt, water, sugar, fats and oils. While it is true, most households will use these ingredients at home, it is highly unlikely we'd use them in the quantities found in the products from the supermarket. Not to mention, we may choose better quality versions of these ingredients than manufacturers.

About Ultra Processed Foods

If we look to the NOVA Food Classification System used overseas, most packet lunchbox foods fall into the category of **Ultra-Processed Foods,** which are defined as "... industrial formulations typically with five or more, and usually many ingredients."[28]

If we look to the Brazilian Food and Nutrition Guide, this is what it says:

"Avoid ultra-processed products. Because of their ingredients, ultra-processed products – such as packaged snacks, soft drinks, and instant noodles – are nutritionally unbalanced. As a result of their formulation and presentation, they tend to be consumed in excess, and displace natural or minimally processed foods. Their means of production, distribution, marketing, and consumption damage culture, social life, and the environment."[29]

That is a strong and pertinent statement from the Brazilian guide and is an accurate summary of what has happened in Australia, to lunchbox foods.

At the time of writing this book, several stories broke in the media following the release of results of a number of studies showing the negative impacts Ultra-Processed Food is having on our health. Headlines like:

- Ultra-processed food linked to early death – BBC News, 30 May 2019
- Processed foods make us fatter, lead to cancer, and are linked with early death. But what exactly is a processed food? – Business Insider, 18 May 2019
- Just four servings of ultra-processed food a day is still too much – Sydney Morning Herald, 30 May 2019
- Ultra-processed food link to disease and death grows — so do we need to shift our food policy? – ABC News, 30 May 2019

It is great to finally see this making headlines. I found the following quote from the article in the Sydney Morning Herald very interesting.

"The authors (of the study) point out that the cumulative and cocktail effects of eating different processed foods 'remain largely unknown'. They suggest that certain food additives may adversely affect cardiovascular health and that certain processing techniques may also be having a detrimental effect on our health."

JOURNALIST, SARAH BARRY

As a busy parent, it is hard to compete with the marketing of the convenient lunchbox products. Some of it is clearly directed at the kids with the cute characters, colourful and artistic letters. They direct other aspects at us adults reminding us how busy we are, how convenient the packets are and therefore we need these products to make our life easier. Once your kids taste them, they are quickly and easily influenced by the tastes because they're scientifically designed to create a taste that makes our kids want to keep coming back to them. Even if you don't buy them, they will taste them at school when their friends give them some. I know it is hard as a parent to say "no", but once you determine your family's health is a priority, you can start taking action to reduce these products from your life.

Cooking Food vs Manufacturing Food

If you have a spare twenty-six minutes, I strongly encourage you to watch Michael Pollan's talk on "How Cooking Can Change Your Life"[30]. He explains how the industrialisation of food came to be and gives you a great understanding of how health has changed since we've stopped eating homemade food and swapped it for industrialised food.

At home when we cook, we chop, slice, dice, mince, blend, sauté, boil, simmer etc. Industrialised food processing is food made in a factory using processes such as liquification, emulsification, pasteurisation, chemical extraction, macerating, hydrogenation, grilling, frying and other cooking methods, and much more. This is mostly managed by sophisticated machinery.

Before food made in a factory became big, the ingredients we used to cook with in our own kitchens were whole foods—single ingredients close to their natural state. Now days, factory-made foods fill the average pantry. Bottled sauces, packet mixes, sachets, boxed foods and more. Factory-made food primarily uses ingredients that are not whole foods nor close to their original source of origin. The ingredients might be derived from plants, animals, synthetic sources, petroleum and more.

When we shop for our groceries, we usually have a budget and we try to stretch it as far as it can go. Our motive is to feed our family the best way we can. Food manufacturers do this on a much bigger scale, but their motives are different. They provide food choices people buy so they subsequently make a profit for their business.

Your family or their health is unlikely to be a big part of the consideration of Big Business in choosing the ingredients or the processing methods used by food manufacturers.

Over the years, there has been a lot of discussion about the impact of salt on health and more recently the impact of sugar on health. You will have read about this from Jo Atkinson in the previous chapter.

Sugar was hotly discussed at the recent Senate Select Committee into the Obesity Epidemic. The negative impacts on health, from the overconsumption of salt and sugar is significant and we must no longer take it lightly. However, after visiting over 100 schools and talking to thousands of teachers, I strongly believe it is time to bring additives and preservatives under the spotlight too.

I have repeatedly heard teachers talk about the time spent managing behaviour in a classroom. The stress they are under to fulfil the requirements of curriculum in these circumstances is a real eye opener. Children today are eating processed, packaged foods at home for breakfast, at school in their lunchbox, at home for afternoon tea and it's probable their evening meals include sauces and the like made in a factory. Our children are literally eating industrialised food all day. We believe, and this is supported by many scientific studies, the ingredients of these foods are having an impact in the classroom and affecting teacher stress levels.

For years, the Food Intolerance Network has been trying to spread the message about how additives and preservatives can be harmful to health. Their website documents case study after case study of children who are affected adversely by additives and preservatives. Children who have skin ailments, behavioural issues, asthma and more.

From time to time on The Root Cause social media pages we share information about products and what's in them. We receive loads of supporting comments from parents sharing their stories of how their children are affected by some additives and preservatives. These posts also come with their fair share of aggressive comments from people who think this information is rubbish and we're taking away children's fun, or worse, we're ruining their childhood! Everyone has their own journey, and for these people, their journey hasn't started and that's okay. My journey began when I realised the impact of packaged, convenient foods were having on the health of my daughter and my husband. I've also seen the change that came to our family from my returning to the kitchen and cooking more foods from scratch. Additives, preservatives, added sugar and added salt I know is harmful to health. My mission is to inform those who wish to be informed in order to preserve and maintain the health of their family.

Francine Bell from Additive Free Kids is one of Australia's

leading experts in Additives. She is an Additive Free Food Coach and Consultant, and an Advisor to the Global Anti Additive Organisation. Francine contributed the remainder of this chapter and the entire next chapter, and shares what you need to know about the labelling on packets and about what you need to look out for as an ingredient detective (i.e. when you ask, "What's In My Food?").

The Rise of Processed Foods

"Six out of ten Australian packaged foods are highly or ultra-processed. More than half are discretionary/junk foods and only one third are healthy."[31] These are shocking statistics. Our children need better choices!

The rise of industrial food processing in the late 19th century thanks to transportation, refrigeration technology, increasing urbanisation and the like, have resulted in many routines and procedures like home cooking becoming obsolete. The proliferation of convenience foods has caused a disconnect for consumers in understanding where their foods have come from and how to use them.

Have you noticed how long the ingredient lists are on packaged food?! In the past, the ingredient list would be only a few lines long and the ingredients recognisable. When I say recognisable, I mean we knew what they were. We used to have the same ingredients in our own pantry or our grandmother's pantry.

Not anymore. You will often find long ingredients listed including ingredients such as: vegetable oils, a multitude of sugars, colours, flavours, preservatives and a host of other additives.

Many of these ingredients sound like a laboratory experiment. We have no idea what they are. Truth be told, some manufacturers don't know what they are either because they buy them from other suppliers! More on this a little later.

There are a few things we need to understand regarding our food regulatory system.

How Does Food Labelling Work in Australia?

Food Standards Australia New Zealand (FSANZ) governs the use of ingredients (including processing aids, colourings, additives, vitamins and minerals) in our food. They also are responsible for some requirements around labelling of our foods. They have a user guide "Ingredient labelling of foods" which discusses:

- Basics of ingredient labelling
- Use of generic names
- Exemptions from ingredient labelling
- Mandatory statements and declarations
- Compound ingredients
- Declaring specific ingredients
- Percentage labelling and characterising ingredients

FSANZ require an ingredient which is "any substance, including a food additive, used in the preparation, manufacture or handling of a food" must be listed in the statement of ingredients.

Sounds simple enough but let's look at how it gets complicated.

They must declare ingredients using one of the following:
- The common name of the ingredient
- A name that describes the true nature of the ingredient
- A generic name of the ingredient (for example spices, sugar, fruit)

So, if a product contained fruit, say apples and pears, they could display it in the ingredients list as:

- Fruit or
- Fruit (apple, pear)

Compound ingredients

Where an ingredient is made from two or more ingredients, for example spaghetti (flour, egg and water) it needs to be disclosed as either:

- Spaghetti (flour, egg and water) or
- Flour, egg, water

Now here is the tricky bit. If the compound ingredient is less than 5% of the food, it does not need to be disclosed at all. And if it is over 5%, then it only needs to be declared if it is a food additive that performs a technological function. It should be noted that is an ingredient that makes up a compound ingredient is a known allergen; it must be disclosed regardless of how much is used. There is a long list of what ingredients form a technological function. These are:

• Acidity regulator	• Anti-caking agent	• Antioxidant
• Bulking agent	• Colouring	• Emulsifier
• Firming agent	• Flavour enhancer	• Flavouring
• Foaming agent	• Gelling agent	• Glazing agent
• Humectant	• Intense sweetener	• Preservative
• Propellant	• Raising agent	• Sequestrant
• Stabiliser	• Thickener	

A good example to understand this is antioxidants in vegetable oils. This antioxidant may not be performing a technological function once they've added it to a biscuit then baked it.

But there are even exceptions to this 5% rule, meaning there are ingredients that do not even need to be disclosed at all.

Two of these I would like to draw your attention to are processing aids and flavours.

1. Processing aids

These are ingredients added to food during processing that may be removed before it reaches its finished form. Or may stay present in the food but deemed to be at an insignificant level and have no effect on the finished food. Or where they are converted to components that occur naturally in food at insignificant levels.

2. Ingredients of flavourings

Manufacturers are required to declare the flavourings used but not the ingredients used to make the flavourings. When you see the word flavour (artificial or natural) this isn't just one ingredient. Usually, this one ingredient can have anywhere from 50-100 ingredients!

The ingredients list is the best indication of what is in a processed food, but it is not definitive because not everything needs to be listed. You will need to keep this in mind if you are trying to be an ingredient detective to see if your child is affected by an ingredient in the food.

What about labels that say No Added... or No Artificial..., No...?

In the true sense of the labelling laws, these are truths. As a consumer, be aware the words No Added or No Artificial should be a red flag. This is all marketing. Turn your packets around and look at the ingredients.

Manufacturers will often play upon the fact consumers see fruit flavours and natural flavours as healthier options. Just because they label a product as strawberry yoghurt, for example, it doesn't mean it contains any strawberries.

What are Additives?

Broadly speaking, you can categorise additives into those ingredients that extend shelf life (such as antioxidants, preservatives, acidity regulators). And those that act on the consistency and sensory qualities of a food (emulsifiers, stabilisers, sweeteners, flavour enhancers, colours).

Some of these additives have negative potential effects when consumed and symptoms can include:

- Learning difficulties
- Behavioural problems
- Hyperactivity
- Headaches
- Asthma
- Skin conditions (like eczema and dermatitis)
- Sleep disturbances
- Anxiety
- Depression
- Allergic and hypersensitive reactions and more

This does not mean all children or adults will be potentially affected, but some will and are.

If a family eats breakfast cereal, has snacks from a packet, eats take out or cooks foods using packets, jars and cans, then it is likely everyday they are consuming some level of additives. For many of this current generation of children, they will have been exposed to additives and preservatives ever since they were babies. This can start in their formula, bottled foods, pouches and so on.

Because we expose children to these ingredients from such a young age, unless you are on the lookout for symptoms and watching what your child is eating, it is possible to think my children aren't affected by additives. From the work I've done, coaching and mentoring clients, many parents are unaware it affects their children until we remove the foods containing these ingredients from what the children are eating. In some cases, it may take only a matter of days before parents see a difference in their child or their own health.

Many parents are unaware additives affect their child
until they remove some or all of them
from the foods they eat.

If It's On the Shelf, It Must Be Safe, Right?

If the product is on the shelf, then it means it should comply with FSANZ food regulations.

FSANZ themselves do not conduct any studies on the actual safety of ingredients. FSANZ undertake a risk assessment where it is the responsibility of the makers of the ingredients to show proof their ingredients are safe.

By now you will understand we have loopholes in our labelling regulations. We need to remember additives are approved on an adult's body mass and they don't test additives in combination, they are tested in isolation. We don't know the full effect of the additives in the processed food our young children are eating. Many additives used here in Australia have already been banned around the world in other countries or are required to be accompanied by a warning label.

Makers of the ingredients assess the safety of additives on an individual basis. To date, there hasn't been any study or assessment done on the safety of foods when multiple additives are combined in one package. This is very common in lunchbox packet foods.

There is so much confusion regarding whether additives are safe as studies are often funded by Big Food Corporations and contrary to independent studies. New science is constantly emerging all the time showing how harmful these additives are.

FSANZ believe only a small percentage of the population is negatively impacted by additives. The reality is we have no idea how big the problem is or how many people it affects.

To this day, there isn't a government-funded agency in Australia to note complaints or reactions regarding food additives. This means there isn't any monitoring of what is in our food at all. Our health is our responsibility.

This means it comes down to each one of us being our own ingredient detectives and actively ask "What's In My Food?" not just once, but continually because companies update their formulations from time to time. Let's look at some to keep your eye out for.

What's the Big Deal With Flavours?

Food manufacturers will purchase flavours from flavour houses (a silent partner in the manufacturing process). They will often provide these flavours in liquid or powder forms. The flavour houses are not obliged to divulge the ingredients of these flavours, not even to their customers—the food manufacturers.

The flavour houses will argue the ingredients are their intellectual property and they are trade secrets. The food labelling laws protect them and their intellectual property from divulging them. This means we have no idea what the flavours are.

Over the years, there has been a lot of talk about how artificial flavours were affecting people, particularly children's behaviour. This led to some flavour houses producing natural flavours for manufacturers to use. We still have no idea what they make them from. To be called "natural", means it must have initially been derived from an animal or plant source.

Are the Natural Flavours Better Than Artificial Flavours?

Natural flavours are flavouring substances obtained by physical processes that may cause unavoidable / unintentional changes in the chemical structure of the flavouring. A variety of methods obtain these flavours including:

- Distillation and solvent extraction
- Enzymatic processes or
- Microbiological processes from plant or animal origin.

So even if the ingredient started as a natural ingredient to begin with, by the end of all the processing and manufacturing, it isn't much different to the synthetic / artificial ones.

Natural flavours is the fourth most common ingredient used in processed food. The only ingredients that come before that are: salt, water and sugar.

Artificial (synthetic) flavouring are flavours derived by chemical synthesis. These flavours are entirely manmade in a chemistry lab.

Whether the flavours claim to be natural or otherwise, they are best avoided.

What Else Should We be Looking Out For in our Food?

Food additives are chemicals that keep foods fresh or enhance their colour, flavour or texture. Additives and processed food go together. The more highly processed the food is, the more additives you are likely to consume.

Most people have the perception that additives must only be in red cordial, coloured lollies, etc. Additives are in EVERYTHING we eat. Even if you aren't giving your kids junk regularly, they may still be eating a huge amount of additives.

Manufacturers add food additives to anything and everything we consume. You will find them in juice boxes, muesli bars, yoghurts, crackers, luncheon meats, drinks, bread and even in medication and personal care products. They are in everything, even the perceived healthier foods.

The key is to understand what they are, how they affect your children and if they are harmful to the human body or not.

What are Some Ingredients You Need to Look Out For?

Food labels can be very daunting and confusing to understand. Often when shopping, we are rushed with small children in tow and don't have time to read the labels properly in the supermarket. Manufacturers should list any substance used to make a food in the statement of ingredients.

You will normally find most additives listed together with other ingredients in the ingredients panel. We often find this near the nutrition information panel on a product. Sometimes the additive is spelled out in full. Other times it is represented by a number.

For example, Cochineal, which is a colour, could be listed as:
* Cochineal
* Colour (120)
* 120

What's the Easiest Way to Avoid Additives?

This is simple. Just eat mainly fresh and only lightly processed foods. This means looking at the ingredients list and choosing those products with the least number of ingredients as your starting point.

One of the biggest challenges for working parents with children is balancing work, life and personal time. Working longer hours, combined with the growing lack of cooking skills or the energy to cook, increases the attractiveness of convenience foods. Occasionally we need some quick options we know are good for our family. They do exist. We just need to know how to find them. That's one reason we are sharing in this book. To help make it easier for you.

Is It Okay to Have Additives Every Now and Again?

By now you have probably realised there is a lot more in processed food than many people realise. I cannot emphasise it enough. You really need to check the ingredients of the packaged food before you buy it and investigate and research more yourself about the additives in the products. If the ingredient(s) has been identified as having negative potential effects and symptoms, then your best course of action is to avoid it. Every dose can do damage. Just because you don't see the damage, doesn't mean it isn't happening. This is like arguing a cigarette now and then is fine. You don't know when the serious adverse reactions will occur.

Do I Have to Spend Hours in the Kitchen Making Everything From Scratch to Avoid Additives?

It is becoming much easier to find great brands and shops that provide simple solutions for us to avoid additives, so we don't need to make it difficult if we don't want to. With some simple planning and preparation, making real food doesn't take that much time and the end result is so much better for you. What we require first and foremost is a change in mindset and attitude, not more time or money.

Additive Free Kids has launched its endorsement program which will provide an independent assessment and review of products on behalf of the community. Consumers can then shop with confidence, knowing each ingredient has been reviewed and screened, saving parents time and giving them peace of mind.

This endorsement program was trialled in some WA IGA supermarkets with great success. The trial showed that when consumers are given the knowledge to help in their decision making process, they will opt for additive free. Additive free stock items flew off the shelves first.

The next step is to have this endorsement on the front of products so that all Australian parents can make the same informed decisions.

The Additive Free Marketplace Directory is another great resource for parents to find additive free products that have been screened on their behalf.

What Advice Can I Offer You?

From one parent to another, the advice I offer you is please take responsibility for your own children's health. Make it an everyday practice of asking "What's In My Food?" whenever you are buying packet foods.

The government isn't planning on removing these additives from our food supply any time soon. We have seen in recent times how hard it is to get change when it comes to sugar and getting clarity with how much added sugar there exactly is in an ingredient. From all accounts, despite The Root Cause raising additives and preservatives as an issue with the recent Senate Select Committee into the Obesity Epidemic, looking at additives and preservatives did not feature in any of the recommendations in the Committee's report.

We have a right to know what is in our food. We have a responsibility to know what we are feeding our young ones and if we are giving them the best possible chance to grow and thrive. Together, we can make change by voting with our dollar for the world we want to see each time we visit the supermarket. We have the power.

Francine's tips for you are:
- Make sure you disregard any claims on the front of pack labels.
- Please make sure you turn the pack over and head straight to the ingredient list.
- If you don't know the ingredients, or you don't cook with them yourself, put the product back on the shelf.

Chapter 6
The 6 Most Problematic Additives

Following on from the previous chapter about the Industrialisation of Food, Francine Bell had so much more detail to add about the most problematic additives in foods, and their effects, that it deserved its own chapter. This chapter is also contributed by Francine.

The 6 Most Problematic Additives are:
1. Flavour enhancers (600 numbers) and flavours
2. Food colourings (100 numbers)
3. Preservatives (200 numbers)
4. Antioxidants (300 numbers)
5. Artificial sweeteners (900 numbers and 420)
6. Emulsifiers

1. What are Flavour Enhancers (600 numbers) and Flavours?

Flavour enhancers add flavour or enhance the power of a flavour.

One of the big flavour enhancers we want to avoid is MSG. Many people believe MSG is a preservative. It isn't. It is a flavour enhancer. MSG will boost the flavour of almost any food.

In the early 1900s, the Japanese isolated and identified the chemical component (glutamic acid) in seaweed when combined with sodium produced a strong seasoning. Mono Sodium Glutamate (MSG) was created and a patent granted in 1909. By 1933, the Japanese were producing 10 million pounds annually. Americans weren't convinced to use MSG widely until 1948. Today Americans alone consume 80 million pounds of MSG a year. That's over 36 million kilograms!

Food manufacturers use MSG as it adds a unique flavour to their product. It removes bitterness and the metallic taste of canned foods.

When you consume MSG, it causes the taste sensation to spread throughout the mouth giving food a fuller flavour by exposing the food to all the taste buds. MSG is popular with food manufacturers because it enhances the flavour so much that less of the expensive foods like meat and spices need to be added to the product. This makes for cheaper production.

MSG is a classic example of how food manufacturing changes evolve. The Japanese originally made MSG from seaweed. Today manufacturers produce MSG from any animal or protein source by using processes such as: hyrdrolysing, extracting and isolating.

The additive number for MSG is 621. Today with the sophistication of food science, food technology and processing methods, manufacturers can produce flavour enhancers which serve the same purpose and have the same effects on the body as MSG. For ease of reading this book, we will call these MSG equivalents by the same name: MSG.

You will find flavour enhancers in the 600 range of numbers and starting from 620 until 641 series. I recommend avoiding all 600 numbers.

What are the effects of MSG?

MSG goes through the digestive system process and is absorbed into the bloodstream. Studies have shown glutamate is a nerve toxin and it can cause nerves to swell as soon as it makes contact. MSG is an excitotoxin, causing the brain cells to over excite and die either immediately or within a few hours. This can cause damage throughout the brain and central nervous system.

Effects are numerous from:
- Neurological disorders
- Pain
- Digestive upsets
- Loss of memory
- Lack of concentration
- Headaches
- Shoulder pain
- Asthma
- Mood changes
- Anxiety attacks

These effects can occur with just occasional exposure for those who are sensitive to MSG. Those who are extremely sensitive may get sore tummy straight after consuming MSG. Some people are allergic to it and break out in hives, rashes or swelling. Some people react with symptoms that look like heart attacks. Other people can also have neck, back or joint pain because of MSG.

Similar to other toxins such as alcohol and the like, MSG is a toxin that is dose dependant. A little alcohol may make you merry, a lot more can make you throw up and pass out, too much can kill you. MSG will cause a reaction in anybody if the dose is large enough. This dose is cumulative too. It's not just what's eaten today, it adds up when consumed regularly. Some people are more sensitive than others.

People often say they feel so much better when MSG has been removed from their diet. They report examples ranging from:

- More energy
- Less temperamental
- Memory is better
- It improves comprehension
- More optimistic.

Some common reactions to keep an eye out for in our children include:

- Poor performance in school
- Lack of concentration
- Behavioural problems
- Learning difficulties
- Stomach upsets
- Headaches
- Asthma
- Sleep disturbances

It's easy to see how this is possible. Young kids are most at risk because the blood brain barrier isn't fully developed during childhood. What is concerning, is many lunchbox packet foods containing flavours, contain these MSG equivalent ingredients.

You will find MSG in packaged foods, processed foods, snack foods, frozen dinners, processed meats, canned and dry soup, stocks, restaurant food and sometimes even vitamins. You really need to turn that packet around, find the ingredients list and look at the numbers or even for words you don't recognise as ingredients you have in your own pantry.

Can MSG be hidden in our foods?

The answer is yes, MSG can disguised in many ways. You will often find claims:

"No Added MSG"

"All Natural"

Or you may find:

"No Preservatives"

"No Artificial Colours"

"No Artificial Flavours"

Whilst this is technically correct and legal, what the manufacturers are doing is advertising by omission. What they aren't drawing your attention to is the fact the product contains flavour enhancers and sometimes multiple flavour enhancers. Let's look at an example:

Looking at a packet of Mamee Monster Noodle Snacks, Chicken Flavour. On the front of the packet it says, "No Added MSG".

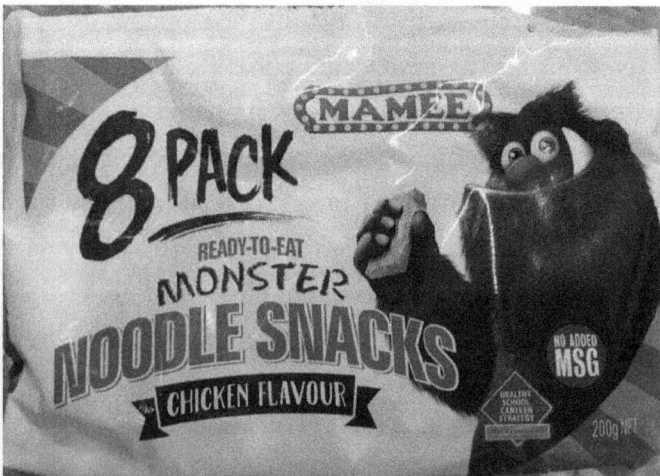

Now turn the packet over and look at the ingredients. As we know,

MSG, or Monosodium glutamate would be listed as number 621. We can see this packet doesn't contain 621, but we can see it contains:

627 - Disodium 5 – guanylate and
631 - Disodium 5' – inosinate

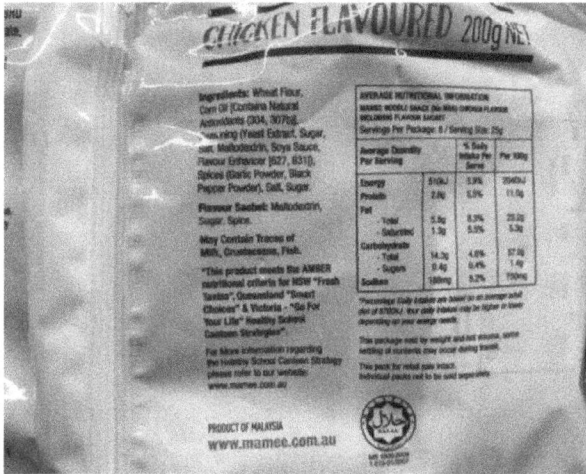

So technically these aren't MSG, but they are flavour enhancers that have the same effect as MSG. Always ignore the front of pack claims. Flip the packet over and read the ingredients list. Avoid all flavours (natural or artificial). Labelling loopholes have allowed manufacturers to hide the use of ingredients that produce the same effects as MSG. At the back of this book, you will find a table listing the many ingredients which can have the same effects as MSG but allow claims of "No Added MSG" to be used.

Every time I've contacted a manufacturer regarding what is included in their flavours, the response is often: "that is proprietary information" and / or "we buy that flavouring in from a supplier".

So, even if it doesn't contain MSG, it often contains too many ingredients that can't fit on a label. Or it's been produced in a laboratory or has been through a thoroughly over processed / extraction process. It is safer to avoid.

2. What About Food Colours (100 numbers)?

Food colouring is any dye, pigment or substance that imparts colour when added to food or drink. Manufacturers include food colouring in many foods, and in places we wouldn't expect – like vanilla yoghurt. You will know an additive is a food colouring if the ingredients list includes ingredients in the 100 series of numbers.

They use food colouring in food for many reasons:

- Extreme temperatures, moisture, storage conditions or exposure to light can overprocess food and as a result they can lose colour.
- Natural variations occur in food generally and sometimes colouring is used to correct the variations and ensure uniformity across the product.
- You will find natural colours are often not as vibrant as compared to what the consumers are used to seeing, so food colouring can boost the colour.
- Some foods that have been over processed are often colourless and bland. By adding food colouring, they add fun back into the product.
- Brightly coloured food looks more appealing, especially to young children!
- Also, food colouring can be used for a practical person in terms of identification for flavours or medicine dosage.

There are five sources that food colouring can be derived from: plant; synthetic / petroleum; animal / insect; minerals; or Nano technology.

Natural ingredients are derived from natural sources (i.e. beets provide beet powder used as food colouring). Other ingredients are not found in nature and therefore must be synthetically produced as artificial ingredients.

Some ingredients found in nature can be manufactured artificially and produced more economically, with greater clarity and more consistent quality, than their natural counterparts. For example, Vitamin C may be derived from an orange or produced in a laboratory.[32]

A growing number of natural food colourings are being produced because of concerns surrounding artificial colourings. We still need to be careful. "Natural" food colourings are still made in a chemistry lab and can still cause allergic reactions and anaphylactic shock in sensitive individuals. Typical examples include: Annatto extracts (160b), Cochineal and Carmine (120).

- Annatto (160b) gives food a yellow to pink colour; common in ice cream and dairy products; potential effects and symptoms include head banging, headache, behavioural problems, hyperactivity, skin ailments and sleep disturbance.
- Cochineal and Carmine (120) colours food red; common in bakery foods, biscuits, lollies, candy canes; potential effects and symptoms include anaphylaxis, asthma, rashes, hayfever, hyperactivity, and skin ailments like eczema.

3. What's the Fuss About Preservatives (200 numbers)?

Preservatives do serve an important function. They are used to keep products fresher for longer and stop microbes from multiplying and spoiling the food. Preservatives have been used since prehistoric times. They made the difference between starvation and surviving a long winter. How foods have been preserved has evolved over the centuries and has been very important to our food security.[33]

Preservatives other than the natural oil, salt and sugar began in the late 19th century, and became widespread in the 20th century. They are now becoming more widespread and used in many more foods than they used to be.

Today the foods in our supermarket travel long food miles.

They are manufactured far away from where the products are sold. Preservatives are added so these products can travel a long distance from the plant to your pantry and then still be fresh when you open the product at home. Preservatives are used to extend the food's shelf life. Many of the foods we buy, if they didn't contain preservatives, could cause food-borne illnesses such as food poisoning.

Preservatives can be natural or manmade chemicals. They can be added to foods, drinks, medicines or cosmetics. They can take two forms – Physical or Chemical. Physical preservation includes processes such as refrigeration, drying or dehydration, freezing, using salt or sugar, alcohol and vinegar. Chemical preservative involves adding chemical additives to the product and include Sorbates, Benzoates, Sulphites, Propionates, Nitrates.

There are serious issues that can be caused by ingesting some preservatives. Often reactions to preservatives do not show straight away as they might with colours. Reactions can be delayed, and this can make it hard to identify. Some preservatives are dangerous for those with asthma whilst others can cause learning difficulties, and behavioural problems in our children.

You will find preservatives in the 200 range of numbers. Some potential effects and symptoms for preservatives in this range include:
- Asthma
- Headaches and migraines
- Dizziness
- Stomach upset
- Skin ailments such as eczema and dermatitis

One of the most common preservatives are sulphites. Sulphur compounds have been used by the ancient Greeks and Romans for centuries to preserve wine. Sulphites are still used today in wineries to destroy bacteria in wine storage vats. Sulphites can trigger wheezing and throat tightening for those who are sensitive and in some asthma patients within 1 to 2 minutes of ingesting.

Under the Food Standards Code here in Australia, manufacturers must declare added sulphites in the list of ingredients on the label of packaged food when it is present in concentrations of 10mg/kg or more. This allows consumers who are sensitive to avoid these foods. You will see preservative listed followed by the specific name e.g. sulphur dioxide and the code number i.e. 220.

If the food isn't packaged, i.e. if it's sold in bulk bins, sulphites still need to be declared on or in connection with the display of the food, or the consumer can request this info. You will often find sulphites in dried fruit (dried apricots, dried apple, sultanas), cordials, juice, fruit juice drinks, pickled vegetables (onions, gherkins), sausages, frankfurts, vinegar and wine. It's also commonly applied to fresh grapes.

Another common preservative that manufacturers like to use are nitrates and nitrites (249-252). They add these to foods such as cured meats like bacon and salami to give them colour and prolong their shelf life. They are also used to prevent fats from going rancid and keep bacteria from growing.

Using nitrates in food preservation is controversial. Nitrosamines can form when nitrates are present in high concentrations and they cook the product at high temperatures. Nitrosamines are carcinogenic.

The International Agency for Research on Cancer[34] (IARC), which is part of The World Health Organisation (WHO) has classified processed meats including ham, bacon, salami and frankfurters as a Group 1 carcinogen (known to cause cancer). IARC concluded there was sufficient evidence the consumption of processed meats causes colorectal cancer.

You may have seen a proliferation of nitrate free options hitting supermarket shelves in recent times. A word of warning, nitrate free doesn't always mean additive free. Some butchers are using other additives instead to achieve the same effects, such as celery extracts. The butchers are most likely advised celery extracts are all natural.

While nitrates occur naturally in food such as spinach and celery, and come with their own vitamin C and other compounds that inhibit the conversion into nitrosamines, we need to keep an eye out for cultured celery extracts. Manufacturers create cultured celery extracts in a lab where they combine the plant's juices with bacterial cultures. Products containing these cultured extracts can have as much or more nitrates than foods listed with sodium nitrite.

It is possible to have nitrate free bacon that is also additive free. Your best chance of finding it will be at an organic butcher. Ask your butcher lots of questions and don't be afraid to ask to see the ingredients they use in making the nitrate free meats. The best indicator it is all natural is that the colour will be much darker than the pink you are used to seeing.

4. What About Antioxidants (300 numbers)? Aren't They Good For Us?

As we age, our body creates free radicals, which can damage living cells and our tissues. Antioxidants are important to stopping or limiting the damage that may be caused by the free radicals. They play a significant role in our health as they can control how fast we age by fighting free radicals. So yes, antioxidants are good for us, but we need to be careful we aren't assuming all antioxidants are the same.

Some examples of great natural antioxidants include
- Fruit: fresh berries, blueberries, blackberries, cranberries, raspberries
- Vegetables: fresh organic (if possible) vegetables are the best, especially green leafy ones. These are ideally consumed raw.
- Nuts: pecans, walnuts, hazelnuts (organic and raw)
- Tea: organic green tea

Then there are antioxidants manmade in chemistry labs. These are usually synthetic antioxidants.

Manufacturers will use the term "antioxidants" to their advantage when using them on an ingredients label. They know the consumer will automatically assume antioxidants are good for my health, therefore, it's fine in this product. Some of them are, but not all of them. Some can be very harmful to some people. These are normally the synthetic antioxidants.

Synthetic antioxidants are a food additive used to preserve food for a longer period of time and stop it from going rancid. Antioxidants act as oxygen scavengers. When we have oxygen in our food, it helps bacteria grow and ultimately harm our food. Without these antioxidants additives in our food, the oxidation of unsaturated fats take place rendering a foul smell and discolouration.

The sole purpose of these antioxidants is to delay the oxidation process. Some additives work by combining with oxygen to prevent oxidation. Others prevent oxygen from reacting with the food. As you can see, antioxidants do serve an important purpose, but because they can be synthetic, made in a chemistry lab, like other additives, they can affect some people. Some common symptoms include:

- Digestive issues – nausea, vomiting, stomach pain
- Respiratory problems – asthma and breathing difficulties
- Skin problems – rash, hives, eczema, dermatitis

Synthetic antioxidants are one of the most hidden of all additives. In many cases, these additives aren't always listed on labels thanks to the labelling loopholes which allow items to remain undisclosed if they represent less than 5% of any ingredient.

For example, if the amount of any ingredient (such as vegetable oil) in a product such as bread forms less than 5% of the product, the food additive, such as an antioxidant BHA 320, it doesn't need to be listed if that additive isn't performing a technological function. The problem is, they use these antioxidants everywhere and they accumulate in the body and can cause serious health effects.

There are plenty of safe alternatives, however, they are more expensive. Food manufacturers often use the cheaper substances.

Foods that have fats and oils are most prone to oxidation. If an ingredient label says vegetable oil or an oil such as canola or sunflower, or other fats, unless some safe alternatives are listed on the label, it is likely to contain antioxidants.

Check the ingredients of your pantry. Look at your cooking oil, margarine, mayo, salad dressing, dips, crackers, biscuits, bread, croissants, potato chips, fried food. Unfortunately, because of the 5% labelling loophole, there are many products on the shelves that contain undeclared antioxidants. You may need to call the manufacturer of the product that contains oils or fats in their ingredients to find out for sure. Not everyone has the time to make these enquiries. Additive Free Kids does the hard work for you. You can find the **Additive Free Marketplace Directory**[35] that lists additive free products that have been screened on your behalf. Often there is a long email exchange with the Manufacturer to get to the bottom of whether they have hidden additives in their ingredients. It is unreasonable to expect the average consumer to do this.

5. What About Artificial Sweeteners (900 numbers and 420), Are They Better Than Sugar?

Food manufacturers are very good at finding a need and providing solutions to those needs. In response to a lot of focus on sugar thanks to some popular films such as "That Sugar Film" or the efforts of the "I Quit Sugar" movement, food manufacturers have produced a wide range of products marketed as diet, sugar free or zero sugar, etc. It stands to reason if you remove the sugar or even the fat from a product that was adding taste, then it needs to be replaced by something else. That's where sweeteners come in.

Artificial sweeteners are synthetic sugar substitutes that can be derived from naturally occurring substances. Artificial sweeteners are also known as an intense sweetener because they are many, many times sweeter than regular sugar. From a manufacturers perspective, it requires little to sweeten a food or drink.

Artificial sweeteners are attractive alternatives to sugar because they add virtually no calories to your diet, which is a very appealing marketing message for those looking to lose weight. There is mixed research about whether artificial sweeteners help with weight control or diabetes. Some say they do, others not. One benefit is that they don't contribute to tooth decay and cavities. However, caution is advised as evidence shows artificial sweeteners come with some negative health consequences.

What is Aspartame (NutraSweet, Equal)?

This is the big one we want to keep our eyes open for! Aspartame is odourless, a white crystalline powder derived from two amino acids. It is 200 times sweeter than sugar and often found in frozen desserts, gelatines, drinks and chewing gum. Aspartame isn't heat stable and hence makes it difficult to use in baking. It is more stable in soft drinks. Aspartame doesn't have a bitter aftertaste whereas some other sweeteners do.

There has been a lot of debate surrounding the safety of aspartame and it has been studied extensively since its discovery. Aspartame has been subject to many claims, including links to cancer and complaints of neurological or psychiatric side effects.

For over twenty years, scientists debated the safety of aspartame. There have been reports of corruption surrounding its approval. Most people assume aspartame is only used in diet foods and drinks. Unfortunately, it is finding its way into a lot of our mainstream foods.

Some consider it to be the most dangerous substance added to our food. The range of symptoms and ailments associated with aspartame include:
- Headaches, migraines, dizziness, seizures, numbness
- Rashes, depression, fatigue, irritability, insomnia
- Vision problems, hearing loss, heart palpitations

- Breathing difficulties, slurred speech, tinnitus, vertigo
- Memory loss, joint pain

There is mixed research on whether aspartame is linked to brain cancer. Studies in the past showed it caused brain tumours in rats. Aspartame is a very controversial additive and we will always be able to find science to back up either side of the argument. Despite this controversy surrounding the safety of aspartame, there is no move by our FSANZ to review or limit the use of aspartame.

Aspartame is now becoming more common and prevalent in our foods. We can find it in 6,000[36] products worldwide, including soft drinks, diet products, low sugar products. Diet drinks, NutraSweet, Equal, Diet Coke, Yoplait yoghurt, chewing gum, sweets, desserts, medications, sugar free cough drops and vitamin supplements.

You will find artificial sweeteners in the 900 range of numbers starting from 950 until 968. I recommend avoiding all numbers in the 900 range and opting for natural sweeteners instead (honey, maple, fruit, dates, etc).

6. What Are Emulsifiers (400 numbers)?

You are probably already aware when you place water and oil together and mix them, if you shake vigorously you will see a dispersion of oil droplets in water and vice versa. If the shaking stops, then the oil and water will separate again. However, if you add an emulsifier, the droplets remain dispersed and a stable emulsion is obtained.

Emulsifiers are the chemicals that allow ingredients to stay mixed. Milk is a great natural example of an emulsion where you have a complex mixture of fat droplets suspended in a watery solution.

Emulsifiers are used in baking to help incorporate fat into the dough and to keep the crumb soft and tender. We find emulsifiers in breads, cakes, cake mixes, and pastry. Emulsifiers also help form an emulsion to make mousses, meringues, ice cream, mayonnaise, salad dressings and margarine.

Recent studies suggest emulsifiers have the potential to damage the intestinal barrier leading to inflammation and increasing the risk of chronic disease. In a recent study, it showed two commonly used emulsifiers had a direct negative effect on the gut microbiome.

They found these additives altered the balance of the gut microbiota causing inflammation which has been directly linked to the development of metabolic syndrome[37], obesity, hyperglycaemia, insulin resistance and chronic colitis. These emulsifiers can affect gut health and if you've read the information in Chapter 2 by Jo Atkinson, you will know how important gut health is to our health.

You will usually find emulsifiers in the 400 series of numbers (with a few exceptions). I recommend avoiding them all.

Francine Bell
Additive Free Food Coach and Consultant.

As you can see from Francine's two chapters, there is certainly a lot to food science used in manufacturing processed packaged foods. It is far simpler and better for your family's health to focus on eating more real wholefoods and minimising the amount of processed package foods you eat. If you want to eat processed packaged foods, remember to turn the packet around and ask "What's In My Food?"

Chapter 7
Food and The Juggling Act Facing Schools

In our travels around Australia presenting The Mad Food Science Program, we identified some different ways food affects schools. What our kids are eating atf home and at school has become a complex issue for schools. Schools right around Australia are juggling the impact food and drinks have on school and classroom dynamics. Their juggling act is made even more tricky by the messages the schools also gives to students about food.

In a school, children get many messages about food. The curriculum has great messages about making healthy choices, but children observe many other messages about food based on what happens in school, such as at sports carnivals, for rewards and more. It is widely accepted children learn more by what they observe from the adults and institutions in their life. Therefore, it stands to reason that the messages children are getting from schools could be exacerbating the problem of what children see as food suitable for school.

Let's explore the ways food is impacting schools.

Breakfast

In Australia, many children are going to school with insufficient fuel to start their day of learning let alone keep them going until lunch break. This insufficient fuel comes in two ways.

1. No breakfast at all

It was eye opening to discover how many children were coming to school with No Breakfast At All!

Just let that sink in. Children are coming to school after sleeping, when their body has fasted, with no food at all. Can you imagine being a child trying to concentrate or learn with no fuel in their body, or being a teacher dealing trying to educate? As we travelled, we discovered the many complex issues existing in households that play a role in this—finances, drugs, violence and more.

The findings from a 2013 Census At School report identified 14.8% of children go to school without breakfast.[38] More recent research indicates this is now about 20%. 1 out of every 5 children.

In 2015, Foodbank, Australia's largest food relief organisation, undertook a survey of teachers across Australia to produce a Hunger in the Classroom report. Below are the core statistics from that report.[39]

- 67% of teachers are seeing children come to school hungry.
- 95% of teachers surveyed, believe "coming to school hungry impacts students' abilities to reach their full potential both in and outside of the classroom."
- Teachers estimate the average student who comes to school hungry loses two hours a day of learning time. If this happens

once a week, then that's a whole term of learning time lost over the course of the year.

- 82% of teachers say their workload increases because of hungry students and distracted students in their class.

The data comments on additional impacts on children:
- Becoming lethargic,
- Finding it difficult to concentrate,
- Experiencing learning difficulties and
- Displaying behavioural problems.

Many schools are trying to overcome the issues having no breakfast creates by setting up breakfast clubs for children in need. In 2015-2016, the Victorian Government allocated $13.7 million across a four-year period to allow Foodbank to establish breakfast club programs in 500 schools of need. In their Interim Evaluation Report, it showed 81% of teachers surveyed reported children who attended breakfast club had improvements in their concentration.[40]

Breakfast clubs tend to provide cereal and toast, usually white bread, for breakfast. While these are not the most nutritious start to the day, it is superior to children not having anything to eat at all.

2. Sugar and additive loaded breakfast

On the flipside of those not getting breakfast are those who get breakfast or grab something on the run at school. The Australian Breakfast Cereal Forum report 2014 stated that approx. 40-50% of primary aged children eat breakfast cereal[41]. Consumer Advocacy Group Choice completed a review in 2016 found that 92% of breakfast cereals contained more than 1 teaspoon of sugar alone[42].

Many of these children are starting their day with breakfast cereals loaded with sugar and additives, flavoured milks, drinks dressed up as a breakfast meal (also loaded with sugar and additives), fast food like McDonalds and even energy drinks. These are just some ways children are starting their day before school.

Something is better than nothing, that goes without saying, but imagine what could be available to these children and their teachers if they started their day with a more nutritious breakfast.

Teachers are starting their class time with many students who are ill-equipped to learn, are hungry or who have eaten foods that create an energy slump around the time they start learning.

Bell Times

In most states, they require public schools to have a maximum of 5.5 hours of instruction time and at least forty minutes of breaks. Traditionally, schools have had a shorter twenty-minute recess earlier in the day, followed by a longer 40 - 60 minute lunch break.

Right around Australia, states and territories included, there is no consistent set of bell times. Principals and schools are juggling bell times to find what works best. A newspaper article reported schools were juggling bell times to "curb unruly behaviour... and because children often went without breakfasts and needed to eat something substantial sooner."[43].

Schools are trying to get the best learning outcome for their students. Some juggling that's happening includes:
- Moving lunch to first break, with recess becoming the later break
- Having a short brain break not long after school starts, followed an hour later with recess, then lunch 2 hours later
- Changing the length of times for the breaks
- Making both breaks equal times in length
- Having an eating time, followed by a play time
- Having play time, followed by an eating time

- Some schools start their day earlier or finish later at 3.25 or 3.30pm.

Eating Times

Eating time is different to bell times. It is the amount of time they give children to eat their lunch.

We found in many schools, in the main lunch break, they gave students an eating time, then a play time. Some schools are even trialling playing first, eat second. The allocated eating time varies, and 10-15 minutes of eating time is the most common.

The intention of this policy is coming from the right place. Their intention is to ensure the children eat their lunch rather than just playing. However, inadvertently it has pitched eating time against play time. If a child hasn't eaten their lunch, they are told to pack up what's left and head out to play or given the option to finish eating and have less play time. Now let's be serious, how many children do you think after sitting in a classroom for a few hours, would give up their play time?

The time allocated to play time and eating time brings up some questions worth pondering:
- What message are the children receiving about the importance of the food they eat?
- Should eating really be rushed?
- Are our kids digesting their food properly?
- Is the speed at which we children are being asked to eat impacting their gut health?
- Are children getting the message; "my food is important because it nourishes my body and brain and helps me to learn," or is it just "I need to eat this quickly so I can go and play?"

We have spoken to many parents and have heard their concerns about the small amount of time children are given to eat. Some have told us they have had to adjust what they pack so they make sure their child will get enough to eat in those 10 or 15 minutes. Others have said they just put packets in because they know their kids can eat it in the given time. Many have commented about food coming home uneaten because the children haven't had enough time to eat.

Could this small window of time to eat also be affecting what children eat from the contents of their lunchbox? We believe so. In The Real Food Lunchbox Project conducted in conjunction with a whole school, we discovered children prioritised their packet lunchbox food first over their main lunch or any fruit or vegetables packed. It was not uncommon for children to have eaten their packet foods first, then made a start on their "real lunch" of a sandwich only to leave it partially uneaten.

Packet foods are specifically designed to get our taste buds excited. Sandwiches, fruit and vegetables don't get these kinds of responses, especially if children are used to eating the flavours of packets. Other food just doesn't taste as delicious. The Real Food Lunchbox study showed when you include processed packet foods in your child's lunchbox, you can expect them to eat those foods and usually first.

If you want your child to eat a nourishing lunch of a sandwich, some vegetables and fruit, you need to minimise the packets so there is more chance of them eating that nourishing lunch.
It is as simple as that.

Brain Break Initiatives

Many schools have also introduced a shorter brain break initiative such as Crunch&Sip® or Munch n Move. These breaks usually happen not long after the bell goes to start the day or after about one hour of classes. The breaks are designed to recognise some children may not have eaten breakfast, or it's been a few hours since breakfast for those who have eaten. Having a little break with fruit or vegetables helps to keep them going until their first longer food break.

In many schools we visited, parents and teachers often referred to these breaks as fruit breaks. Vegetables were not mentioned. In schools which have these initiatives, teachers will often tell you parents believe they do not need to pack more fruits and vegetables because they have included it for this initiative. Data collected from 35 schools who have partnered with us and completed a Food and Waste Survey shows the consumption of vegetables in lunchboxes is less than half a serve of vegetables per lunchbox.

In a 2012 Qualitative Investigation Report of Crunch&Sip® for WA reported on the benefits from the program. The list of benefits reinforce and confirm the importance of children needing fuel in the form of real food to help them learn. The benefits included:

- Reinforced health messages learnt in class.
- Increased consumption of whole foods and "displaced" junk foods being eaten.
- Increased amount of physical activity time for children at recess. What's not clear is whether this meant children did not eat recess because of Crunch&Sip®.
- Improved concentration in class.
- Some schools believed it led to lower levels of hyperactivity because it reduced the number of additives in processed foods because children weren't eating as many processed foods.

The report also shared the results of a survey conducted with school principals.

"Perhaps the foremost conclusion from the present data is that nutrition programs are viewed as non-core school business in contrast to physical activity programs. From a strategic viewpoint, this presents a clear direction for Crunch&Sip®. The assumption schools should place greater value on physical activity than nutrition should be challenged in a long-term program of social and political engineering and advocacy."[44] – Dr Owen Carter and Tina Phan.

These results are consistent with our experience of travelling Australia and encouraging schools to undertake The Mad Food Science Program. We focus on empowering children to eat more fruit and vegetables and minimising processed, packaged foods.

Anecdotally, it would appear many principals are yet to draw a strong enough connection between food and children's performance at school. Perhaps this is also because there is little discussion about this from a government perspective either. In talking about health for instance, most of the government focus is on physical activity initiatives or school canteen. What we know from the 35 schools who have participated in our Food and Waste Survey is across 343 classes, 88% of lunches at school are being sent from home. Not tackling lunchbox food means a big chunk of what may be driving student learning, behaviour and health is not being addressed.

Class and School Rewards

Over the last four years, I have had so many parents express concern about food rewards children receive at school. Some states and schools have policies which specifically state lollies are not to be used as rewards, yet parents still say it occurs. It is a problem. Some schools even have behaviour rewards at a whole school level where children are recognised for good behaviour and are awarded vouchers for "treats" like Zooper Doopers. Let's just have a look at one of these, and ask yourself, is this really a treat if it doesn't help a child's body or their learning? What messages is it sending to the children about food and rewards?

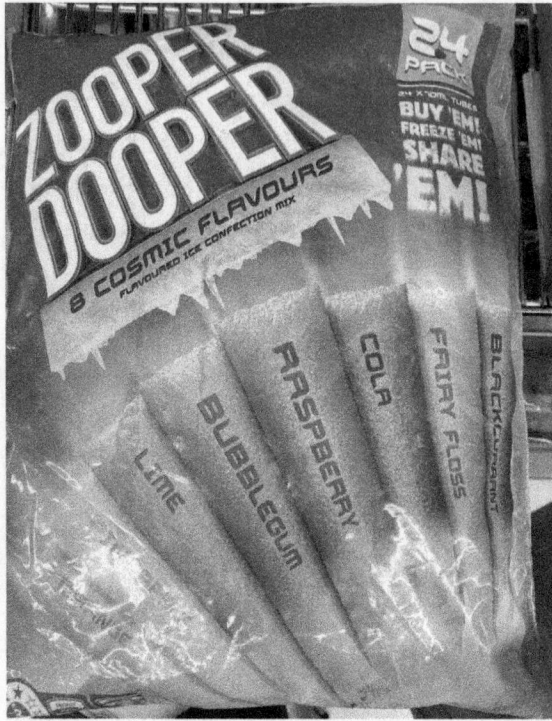

Zooper Dooper Cosmic Flavours are described on the pack as Flavoured Ice Confection Mix. According to the Oxford Dictionary "confection" means "an elaborate sweet dish or delicacy".

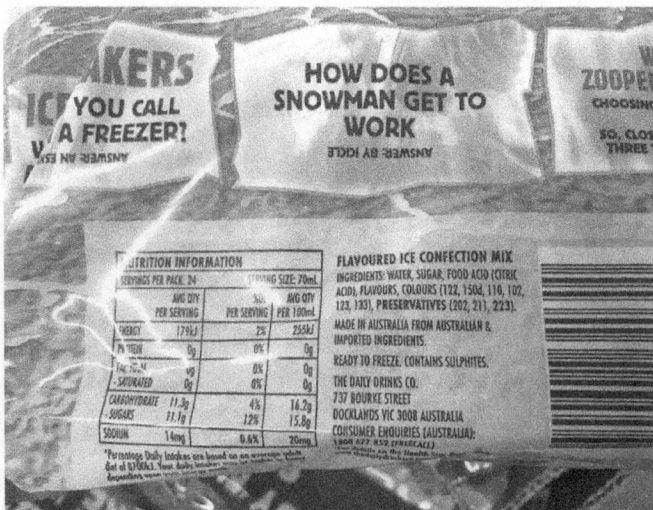

Nutrition Information Panel:

Per serving of Zooper Dooper (1 ice block), there is no protein or fat, but 11.1g of sugar and 14mg salt. This means each Zooper Dooper contains 2.8 teaspoons of sugar!

The World Health Organisation recommends added or free sugars should not be more than 5% of our daily calorie requirements which means for most primary aged kids, this is between 3 and 5 teaspoons. This means one Zooper Dooper is giving primary aged children almost all of the free sugar allocation for the day!

Ingredients:

Water, sugar, food acids (citric acid), flavours, colours (122, 150d, 110, 102, 123, 133), Preservatives (202, 211, 223).

- Water is the main ingredient. That's a good thing.
- Sugar is the next main ingredient. That's not a good thing – 2.8 teaspoons of sugar!
- Food Acids are generally used to enhance the taste in soft drinks and sweets and to create the conditions for the formation of confectionary
- "Flavours" can be made up of 5 to 50 different ingredients. This is like their "secret sauce" so other people or manufacturers can't copy it. Most flavours are modelled off the flavour of an actual food stuff but it's just an imitation of the flavour of that food. So I'm sorry, I can't enlighten you with what's actually in these flavours.

Using the Chemical Maze App, here's what I can share with you about these colours:

- **Colour 122** is also known as Azorubine or Carmoisine. It is banned in USA, Japan and Canada and maybe petroleum derived. In the EU, foods with this colour must carry a health warning. The function of this colour is to make the food look red. It's potential effects and symptoms include Asthma, Hyperactivity, may cause allergic reactions, tantrums, skin ailments such as eczema, dermatitis, itching, hives, rashes etc

- **Colour 150d** is also known as Caramel IV. It may be genetically modified. Potential effects and symptoms include Asthma, gastrointestinal ailments, allergic and hypersensitive reactions and hyperactivity.

- **Colour 110** is also known as Sunset Yellow FCF (sounds pretty eh?). Product labels in the EU must carry a healthy warning. Potential effects and symptoms include Asthma, diarrhoea, hay fever, hyperactivity, nausea, nettle rash or hives, vomiting, behavioural problems, learning difficulties, skin ailments (eczema, dermatitis etc)

- **Colour 102** also known as Tartrazine. Product labels in the EU must carry a healthy warning, Synthetic Azo Dye. Potential effects and symptoms include aggressive behaviour, behavioural problems, difficult concentration, headache, insomnia, learning difficulties, skin rash, suspected musculoskeletal and neurotoxicity, Confusion, depression, hayfever, migraines, hyperactivity, sleep disturbance.

- **Colour 123** also known as Amaranth – not the grain, but the synthetic chemical. Banned in the USA, may be petroleum derived, synthetic azo dye. Potential effects and symptoms include Asthma, gastrointestinal symptoms, may affect liver and kidney function, may cause hyperactivity, skin rash, suspected animal carcinogen, suspected teratogen (which means may be a factor which cause malformation of an embryo), allergic and hypersensitive reactions, hayfever, skin ailments (eczema, dermatitis etc)

- **Colour 133** known as Brilliant Blue, this colour is petroleum derived and a synthetic azo dye. Potential effects and symptoms include allergic reactions, asthma, gastrointestinal symptoms, may cause hyperactivity, rhinitis, suspected carcinogen, suspected mutagen, suspected neurotoxicity, nettle rash or hives, skin ailments (eczema, dermatitis etc).

- **Preservative 202** is also known as Potassium Sorbate. It's mainly petroleum derived. Potential effects and symptoms include allergic reactions, asthma, headache, hyperactivity, skin irritations, behavioural problems.
- **Preservative 211** known as Sodium Benzoate. Petroleum derived. Potential effects and symptoms include asthma, headache, hyperactivity, may damage DNA in cells, skin irritation, stomach upset, hyperactivity, learning difficulties, skin ailments.
- **Preservative 223** Sodium metabisulphite, is synthetically derived. Potential effects and symptoms include hayfever, asthma, suspected respiratory, kidney and immunotoxicity, gastrointestinal ailments, headache, migraine, hyperactivity, skin ailments (eczema, dermatitis etc).

Please be aware, the new No Sugar Zooper Doopers contain flavours, the same colours and preservatives as this version of Zooper Doopers. . The sugar has just been replaced with sweeteners.

I realise ice blocks are considered fun for children, but this sort of chemical concoction are not a healthy choice and are unlikely to support learning.

I like to remind parents when we send our kids to school, we are outsourcing every aspect of our children for the day. The mixture of computer / tv screens, video games, quality of food, lack of sleep and general household issues are all brought to school by our kids. Our teachers are on the receiving end of that but 20+ fold, depending on the number of students in the class. The teachers are dealing with it daily. For teachers, it is a juggling act as to what will achieve the results required for their class. Treats as rewards help get results.

With that in mind, this topic is challenging for me to write because some teachers do use junk foods—lollies, ice blocks, pizzas and more as rewards for their students. Teachers do an amazing job and I can see why they need and choose to reward students. The problem is using food as rewards sends many messages, and mixed messages, to children that food is a reward.

Food rewards can:
- Encourage children to eat sweet foods when they are not even hungry
- Send and create life-long messages for children about using food to comfort or reward themselves
- Make kids desire more sweets
- Affect the normal hunger cues

Research shows we generally create food habits in early childhood. Psychologically using foods as rewards can lead to emotional eating later in life. We need to be educating children on how to manage their appetite. To eat when they are hungry, stop when they are full. Not to eat a sweet "treat" for doing or behaving well.

The short-term impacts of offering food as a reward may seem harmless, but the long-term impacts can affect children's health and happiness ongoing.

Here are some other ways we can reward children:
- Experience based rewards like extra play time, class time with shoes off
- Stickers, stationery
- Free time to read or use class computers
- Books
- Sit in the teacher's chair for the day
- Be the special helper for the day

If you need to start a conversation with your teacher or school, my suggestion is to go in with solutions similar to those listed above rather than complaints. A teacher's job is hard enough.

Even though I am talking about this from a school and teacher perspective, as parents, we need to remember the same thing. Using food as a reward at home sends the same messages to children as it does when it happens at school.

Fundraisers

There is only so much schools can do with the funding the government issues them. Fundraising is a necessity and allow schools to undertake projects moving the school in a forward direction. The Parenting Committees who are responsible for fundraising should firstly be acknowledged for their effort and what they do for the school. It is with much respect that I write this section because as a parent who has been on a committee, I totally get the time commitment and the juggling act it is to raise money to help the school. However, it would be totally remiss of me not to address the food messages children get from many fundraising initiatives.

Like rewards, fundraisers often use junk foods to raise money. Cake stalls, ice block days, pizza days, sausage sizzle, which commonly goes hand in hand with purchasing a can of fizzy drink or a juice and the list goes on. Again, these are sending messages to children about how these foods are fun. These foods make you feel good momentarily, but this short-term gratification may bring behavioural or health effects within a few hours.

Often parents and children do not connect how they feel later after they have eaten this food. It's forgotten. It should also be said these moments of short-term gratification add to everything else that's already being consumed daily. They may be adding up inside the body and have an effect later in life.

In the past year, I have spent many hours researching ways to raise funds. I've been talking to P&C and P&F members about the issues they face when trying to raise funds. Suffice to say, there are plenty of ways to raise more money than these food-based fundraisers, but they all require one thing: **Volunteers**.

This is the biggest challenge faced by P&C's and P&F's. They do not have enough volunteers to tackle the time it takes to implement some fundraising initiatives that can make more money. For instance, a fundraiser like a Colour Run could net a school at least $20,000 which is the equivalent of say twenty good food fundraisers. However, it takes about fifty hours of volunteer implementation time compared to 2-4 hours for each of the smaller food fundraisers. From a P&C perspective, it's far easier to get a few volunteers for 2-4 hours, rather than getting additional volunteers to implement the much bigger, more profitable initiative. This is one of the juggling acts.

With that said, some P&C's I have spoken to are opting to take the more strategic approach of it's better to have one or two larger fundraisers later in the year. They can plan well in advance and spread all the implementation hours out so it's not such a high workload on the small number of volunteers.

Given the constraints of volunteers, perhaps having fundraisers that have healthy food options is the way forward. We have seen schools moving in this direction despite people believing kids won't eat the healthier food. They do, of course.

If you have concerns about the fundraisers your school undertakes, then I strongly recommend you offer to be on the committee, so you get to be involved in what happens in the school. Always be prepared to put forward alternatives and share why it's so important to not be giving children mixed messages about food.

If you want your school fundraisers to be non-food related, then I suggest one of the best things you can do is get together with some friends and offer to volunteer to undertake a fundraiser that requires more resources.

Sports Events

The curriculum requires schools to promote physical activity. This is usually done through sports events like swimming carnivals, cross country and athletics carnivals. However, at many schools when they are hosting these activities designed to promote physical activity, there are usually canteens or tuckshops or school fundraisers selling food to the kids. The foods that are usually on offer are unhealthy. It is not uncommon for cans of drinks, packets of chips and lolly bags to be on sale too. What is the message that children are getting when they exercise and are then allowed to eat foods that do not help their body?

In addition to this sort of messaging, I have received messages from parents who are horrified with activities designed to be fun for the kids, but which inadvertently promote junk food. For example, throwing Minties into the pool and the children having to dive into retrieve them.

If you take a look around at any sports carnival, you'll probably also find sports or energy drinks. These drinks are loaded with sugar, flavours, colours and other additives.

I played a lot of sport as a kid—running, netball, basketball, high jump, hurdles. Any activity that allowed me to move, I did. Whenever we competed at carnivals or had a time break throughout the game, there would always be a parent, a teacher or coach there with orange mouth guards (oranges cut into small wedges) and water to quench the thirst and rehydrate the body.

Fast forward to today, and at the end of the game it is common for a parent, teacher or coach to approach the team with a bag of snakes, frogs, lolly pops, chips and cans of drink. There are also kids who come equipped with sports type drinks like Gatorade or Powerade drink, that usually contain about nine teaspoons of sugar.

Don't even get me started on the colours included in these drinks. For the record, they derive the blue colour from petroleum. In the Chemical Maze app it is listed as having many potential effects. Many parents and children have fallen for the marketing hype which leads one to believe our kids need these drinks to replace electrolytes lost from playing sport. The truth is the body loses water faster than it loses electrolytes so the best drink for our sporty kids is water.

Reports indicate we lose electrolytes after an hour or more of **intensive exercise where you sweat.** It's only when you are sweating are you losing electrolytes. The temperature of the day can impact how much you sweat too. It is highly questionable about whether these drinks are supporting children who have sporadically participated in races. Unless the children are sweating, it's unlikely they need to replace electrolytes.

If your child does play a lot of sport and sweats a lot, water for hydration is key but you can replace the electrolytes naturally with real foods. Nuts, peanut butter, bananas, tomatoes, leafy greens, and coconut water are just some ways.

And, don't even get me started on the use of high profile athletes to market these drinks!

Many parents also feel children need a sugar hit for energy for sport and believe lollies or sugary drinks are the way to do it. Maddy Hille, Dietitian says, "from a dietetics perspective, a high sugar snack e.g. snakes contains simple sugars that will be very quickly broken down in the body meaning you will initially get a hit of energy, but this will be very short lived." So it's possible that giving them a spike of energy from these lollies could also cause a crash of energy whilst they are playing.

Sports allow our kids to do physical exercise. The good that the physical exercise has done for their bodies is negated by the foods and drinks we give them as a reward for participating or because they believe their body needs it.

Teachers' Eating Habits

Teachers go into teaching out of their love for education and children. Like parents, they want the best for children. When at school, teachers become role models to children they are interacting with throughout the day. It could be on the playground or in the classroom. Children notice closely what teachers do and this includes what they eat and how they talk about food. Like some parents, some teachers are also unaware of what's in the food they're eating or in the food supply. As alluded to by Principal Susan Hilliar at the start of the book, there is a whole generation of teachers who are coming through the system now who have grown up having processed food as their normal food since their late primary, early high school years. They don't know any better.

On our Australian Tour, I have witnessed firsthand the messages teachers are sending to children via their own behaviour around food:

- A teacher brought a can of coke to a Mad Food Science workshop. When a student accidentally knocked it over, the teacher made the child sit out of the green smoothie taste test experiment.
- In another experiment involving the participation from a teacher with the students, we gave the teacher a piece of corn and the student a muesli bar as part of the demonstration. Without knowing what was to be asked of them, the teacher commented, "Oh, can I have the muesli bar?"
- In the same experiment, at a different school, a teacher asked if they could swap their piece of corn for a fruit roll up.
- A teacher facilitating the experiment of showing children how to read packet labels, read the ingredients list in her favourite kind of chips and said to the children she was assisting, "Oh well, I love these, so I am going to keep eating them."
- Teachers arriving to Mad Food Science workshops with cans or bottles of soft drink.
- Teachers on playground duty eating packets of chips or chocolate bars.
- The food eaten in staff rooms is often seen by the students.

As adults, be it parent or teacher, we need to be mindful. What we do and say is noticed by the children. Sometimes the kids will see it or hear it and make a comment. All of the time, messages are being delivered even if we don't realise it.

It is quite common for teachers who participate in The Mad Food Science Program to comment that the program was eye opening for them too. It reminds me this information is as important for adults as it is for the children. There is no judgement here. I always remind myself that I was a forty-year-old mother and wife myself before I learnt to question "What's In My Food?" and I only did that because Israel became sick. If he hadn't, I may well have just kept buying foods without questioning, assuming my family was okay because the products were on the supermarket shelf and must be okay too.

What I am about to say may not make me popular, but my job is to raise awareness:

I believe many teachers, principals and school management are yet to draw the connection between what children eat and the impact it can have on their behaviour and performance. Perhaps they realise but think the whole topic is too hard to tackle. But isn't the health of our kids and their ability to reach their full potential worth tackling?

In an effort to raise more awareness about "What's In My Food?" I created a Teacher Professional Development Program focussing on "The Impact Food Has On Teacher and Student Wellbeing". The goal is to educate teachers about how the food they eat can affect their health and performance as a teacher (and a parent), and about how food can impact what happens in the classroom. Most importantly, the program challenges the adults to think about all the different "food touch points" in their school and how these may send mixed messages to the children. These include lunchboxes, canteen, school and class rewards, parties, fundraisers, etc. I am super excited to say it's working well and schools where the whole teacher community participate are more committed to making change at their school. Here's a comment from a teacher who attended a recent session.

"Thank you. Very informative and challenging, you really 'opened my eyes' to what I am eating but also to the responsibility we have to our students. Keep up the incredible work."

ST PATRICKS PRIMARY SCHOOL TEACHER, MACKSVILLE, NSW.

School Canteens

Canteens are an enormous part of the juggling act for schools, and it's one of the most common areas where we are asked to advise parents, teachers or staff at schools. To do justice to this topic, we've allocated the entire next chapter to School Canteens.

Chapter 8
The Role of the School Canteen

If you turn back the clock thirty years, to order lunch from the canteen was largely a "treat" for children. Thirty years back, most children brought simple lunches from home and processed food wasn't as prevalent as it is today. These were my days at school. A canteen order was so exciting. Sausage rolls, pies, finger buns, a small selection of lollies. There was little talk about the food the canteen sold because it wasn't seen as the main food provider for children for their school days. In addition, thirty years ago, there simply was not the health crisis we have today, where many children are eating excess discretionary (junk foods) daily. They rarely mentioned obesity and diabetes type 2 when talking about children's health. Back then, discretionary foods were considered a treat because we rarely had them.

Today, canteens can be considered Australia's leading take away food outlet for children.[45] With many families having both parents in the workforce or single parent families in the workforce, more families rely on the canteen to provide lunch and or recess for their children. There is a need for school canteens to be offering food which provides sustenance to help children with their learning, mood and behaviour, rather than foods that may reduce their ability to concentrate and learn.

The National Healthy School Canteen Guidelines were created in 2014 following a 6 year project funded by the Australian Government. This was the introduction of a traffic light system
- Green for foods that can always be on the menu
- Amber for foods to select carefully from
- Red are not recommended on the canteen menu

It was pleasing to see these guidelines did make mention of additives most likely to cause problems. However, the guidelines also gives examples on how to identify foods as green and amber and one example of flavoured milk includes an additive the same guidelines have listed as may cause a problem.

A problem does seem to be that each State tends to have their own take on a traffic light system. Many applied a traffic light system and most recently, NSW took a big deviation from the National Guidelines with the NSW Healthy Canteen Strategy.

In 2016, the premier of the NSW State Government put forward a goal to reduce childhood obesity by 5% over ten years. One means for doing this was to introduce a new set of guidelines for NSW canteens. Enter the NSW Healthy Canteen Strategy which moved away from the traffic light model. The new guidelines were to be implemented by the end of 2019.

The guidelines have a few principles, these being:

- ¾ of the menu must be made up of Everyday foods.
- ¼ from Occasional foods. These occasional foods must have a Health Star Rating of 3.5 or above.
- Everyday foods must be more widely marketed / visible than the everyday foods.

They implemented this model with the intention of wanting to make a difference to children's health. However, a few problems exist. The system is based on the Health Star Rating system, which at the time of writing is under scrutiny because the algorithm doesn't specifically recognise added sugars. Personally, I feel another issue is the fact the system doesn't take into account the level of processing or additives in a product.

Another issue with canteen guidelines appears to be that State Health Departments develop the guidelines with input from State Education Departments, but ownership of the guidelines is unclear. In some states, there doesn't appear to be resources in either Department to adequately enforce the guidelines. Enforce is the important word here. Some States have resources within the Department of Health who are have roles that are to support and promote health within schools, but the best these resources can do is talk to powers that be in the schools. The principals may also have to sign off to say their canteen complies. From my chats with various departments and principals, what is not clear is whether there are any actual ramifications for non-compliance.

Questionable Green and Amber Foods

It is quite common for parents and even some teachers to reach out to me to express their concern about some of the foods and drinks that are allowed as "Green" or everyday foods or even as Amber foods. Schools and Canteen Managers are issued with buyers guides, and they assume if the food or drink is in the buyer's guide, then it must be ok. However, there are many examples which are questionable. Here's a few examples. When you're looking at these, I want you to ask yourself if these foods are "school foods," or foods you would expect to see at an amusement park.

Product	Contains
Fruchilla Fruit Cup Slushie	200ml serve – 21.8g sugar = 5 teaspoons of sugar **Blueberry – Colour 133**, petroleum derived **Preservative 202** Both have hyperactivity listed as a potential effect. Source: The Chemical Maze
Breaka Strawberry Milk	300ml serve – 10.4g sugar = 2.6 teaspoons of sugar The labelling does not allow us to differentiate between natural sugar from the milk and added sugar, but sugar is the second ingredient in the ingredients list. **Flavour** – we really don't know what is in this **Colour 120** – Cochineal: allergic and hypersensitive reactions, asthma, hyperactivity, skin ailments like eczema listed as potential symptoms. Source: The Chemical Maze

TNT Sour Ice Red Berry Blast Iceblock 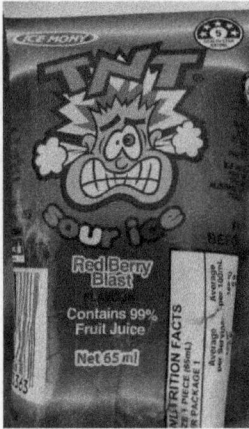	65ml serve – 5g sugar = about 1 tspn sugar **Apple Juice concentrate** is the first ingredient. The World Health Organisation (WHO) deems juice concentrate to be a free (added) sugar. In this one little ice block it is possible for kids to be getting 20-30% of their daily free sugar level as recommended by WHO. **Colour 129 – Allura Red.** Maybe petroleum derived. In the EU foods with this colour must carry a health warning. Potential symptoms include allergic reactions, asthma, behavioural problems, hay fever, hyperactivity, learning difficulties, skin ailments like eczema. Source: The Chemical Maze

Even though Amber (or in NSW occasional) foods are not intended to be eaten every day, the fact they are available on the canteen menu means that some children eat these foods every day.

My message to schools and Canteen Managers is just because a food is in a buyer's guide, does not mean it is healthy and supports learning.

If you are unhappy with what your school is selling at the canteen, the first course of action is to locate your State's canteen guidelines. Compare what is being sold against those guidelines. After you've done this investigation, take your concerns to the principal. It is strongly suggested that you go in with better options rather than just having a complaint. It is likely to be better received. If you are still unhappy with the result, then you can lodge a complaint using the Dept of Education process for your State.

If there is something on the menu that is acceptable in the guidelines, but you strongly believe it does not belong on the menu, follow the same process as above. However, be prepared to show why your school would be better off without the item on the menu. Remind your principal that just because it's green or amber and in the buyer's guide, doesn't mean the school has to buy it.

Just because a food is in a buyers' guide, does not mean you have to buy it. Ask "What's In My Food?" Then work out if you think it will support learning and the health of students.

The Purpose and Ownership of the Canteen

Despite the Healthy Canteen Guidelines being in place, the individual school manages the implementation of the guidelines. The key determinants affecting this management by schools are:

- Is the canteen seen as a profit centre or a community service to the school?
- Who runs the canteen? Is it the school? The P&C/F? Or an outside business the school leases the space to?

Within each of these determinants are other factors at play. For instance, if the canteen is seen as a profit centre by the school, the focus is on selling the items they "believe" children will buy, irrespective of the impact these have on health or classroom behaviour. If it's a community service, then it depends on who has ownership of the running the canteen and their belief about whether the canteen is a treat for kids (some canteen managers still believe this.) –or whether they recognise the canteen needs to offer healthy food that help with learning, growth and development.

In school and P&C/F run canteens, resourcing is a big issue. Volunteers are hard to come by. Many parents are already stressed, time poor and finding time to volunteer or even attend school events is not high on their priority list. Many canteens are run by canteen managers—sometimes volunteer, sometimes paid, but both are as a labour of love. If the school pays the Canteen Manager, many are working way more hours than they are paid for because they love the children.

Canteens run by an outside business face the need for it to be a profitable venture, otherwise it's not a viable business for them. An outside organisation will usually focus on selling products they believe the children will buy and which have a good margin.

Common Myths About Canteens

These issues around canteens are made more complicated by the following two myths that are commonly held either by people in power in the school or the canteen, or the businesses that run the canteens:

1. Kids won't eat healthy food
2. You can't make money selling healthy food.

I refer to these as myths because there are many examples of canteens or tuckshops who are making more money than before by selling healthy real food that the children love. I have showcased some of these canteens on our website. If you want to take a look, jump across to our website www.therootcause.com.au and type in "showcase" into the search bar.

Equipment Obligations

Just when you think the canteen issue couldn't get any more complex, one needs to consider the equipment such as fridges and freezes in canteen facilities. Many school canteens have been "gifted" their fridge and or freezer from a big food company. The usual proviso for keeping the equipment is the canteen must stock a certain number of lines of their product or must order a certain amount of their products regularly.

This becomes an issue for schools who are looking to make their canteens healthier. Suddenly they're being told by big businesses that the school may lose their fridge or freezer unless they keep stocking and ordering sufficient quantities of their products. True story. This means schools may be out of pocket considerably if they choose to opt for healthy options and forgo their "gifted" fridge or freezer.

As you can see, canteen food is a complex issue. Regardless of the guidelines or how the canteen is run, one thing is for sure. The food sold at the canteen is like food in a lunchbox. It needs to nourish a child's body to help their health, their growth, their behaviour and social skills and their ability to learn. As Leanne, the Canteen Manager from Bli Bli State School said, "I am providing food to support an educational environment, not an amusement park."

Successful Canteens

At Point Clare Primary School on the Central Coast of NSW, cordon bleu chef Anwyn Jeannot and the school's P&C have totally transformed the school canteen. All food is now made freshly on site, including sushi rolls and burgers that include grated carrot and zucchini. The new foods have been well received by students, parents and teachers. It also seems to have had a knock on effect because the canteen has a flow of regular volunteers. The school recognises it takes a village to run the canteen.

Canobolas Rural Technology High School in Orange NSW has employed chef Andrew Farley to take over their canteen. Andrew has turned the canteen into a café style operation, serving meals made fresh on site. He's proven even high school kids will choose real food.

Both of these schools have taken their canteens to profits way beyond what the previous pies and sausage rolls style menus achieved. The number of people ordering has increased too. Whilst there is no commentary on whether this has had an impact on learning and behaviour in these schools, what is does support, is that when a school offers healthy options, more people buy them, and real food becomes normal and even cool. If you consider the scientific studies showing children who eat a healthy balanced diets tend to behave and perform better, it is reasonable to expect over the longer term, these schools will reap the benefits of feeding their students nutritious foods.

Chapter 9
The Environmental Impact of Lunchboxes

When we first set off on our Australian Tour, I had not even contemplated the environmental impacts of lunchbox food. I really only got the connection when we ran The Mad Food Science Program at a school in Proserpine. The facilities manager at the school approached me and said, "These kids really need to hear what you have to say. There is so much rubbish at this school." He took me on a tour to show me the two skip bins of rubbish that the school fills almost to the top every week. One was for recyclable rubbish, mainly big cardboard, the other was full of rubbish collected from the school grounds – this was mainly lunchbox rubbish.

I was shocked. I had never correlated that every lunchbox has the potential to create rubbish. I never realised most of this rubbish was not recyclable or if it was, it needed to be separated out and taken somewhere special for processing. Have you thought about this element when packing your child's school lunchbox?

It's pretty safe to say the average lunchbox is creating rubbish, **every single school day.**

Do you realise packaged food like juice or flavoured milk boxes create 3 different types of rubbish? There is the plastic straw, the clear plastic piece that holds the straw and the actual box itself. The facilities manager said these three pieces are often separated out without thinking by children. They pull off the clear plastic to access the straw, drop that, put the straw in, then drink it, then quite often pull the straw out to keep chewing on it, then throw the box away. When the bell goes, the chewed straw is often thrown on the ground. Wow, who would have ever thought about this without being told? This is another good reason why water is the only drink our kids need at school.

He also shared that about half of the waste produced is from partially eaten sandwiches or wraps and whole or partially eaten fruit. Another wow moment. This was the first time I realised children were not eating their lunch and choosing to throw it away instead of taking it home. I asked him for his thoughts about why this is the case. His answer was this:

"I think it's a combination of factors but mostly because they don't get enough time to eat anymore. There's eating time, then there's play time. When eating time is up (i.e. bell rings), whatever is left gets thrown out. Then there's the kids who don't want to eat their real food because everyone else has packets."

This is consistent with what was discovered with The Real Food Lunchbox Project. Children prioritise eating their packet food first and if there's time, they then start to eat their other food—the food we pack because we think it will nourish them. Quite often, the sandwiches and fruit are thrown away partially eaten.

*Lunchbox rubbish is more than just about what kids are eating, it's about what they are **not** eating too.*

From that moment, I adjusted The Mad Food Science Program and its messages to incorporate an element about the environment and the impact our choices make on the planet. We empower children to recognise real food helps their one body for life, and they are so smart that all their scraps can be used, either returned to the earth, fed to chooks, used as compost or even turned into other materials like cups that can biodegrade. The scraps from real food can be reused and help our one planet for life – Earth. Unfortunately, most lunchbox packet foods cannot be reused or if they do, they take significant resources to process into something else.

Reducing Our Environmental Impact

Many schools have wonderful recycling and composting programs which is fabulous, but if most of the rubbish can't be recycled or is costing the planet to recycle them, then we need to rethink what we pack.

One school we visited in Western Australia has developed a fun way of getting their children to really take notice of the rubbish they are creating. They have designed special purple bins for packet waste, and they have been actively showing the children how much waste they are creating. Since implementing the program, the amount of packaged waste has reduced.

Nude Food Days have been great at reducing the amount of waste because they bring focus to the fact lunchbox food creates waste. Some schools have introduced a 100% Nude Food Policy whilst others are doing Nude Food day once a week. Sometimes it is given other names like Trashless Tuesday or Wastefree Wednesday. Some schools have gone so far as removing rubbish bins from their playgrounds and if children bring in rubbish, they have to take it home with them. However, as we discovered from talking to some of these schools, these actions do not necessarily stop children from having processed food in the lunchbox, it just changes the place where the rubbish needs to be dealt with. Packets are opened at home and put into the lunchbox and the rubbish stays at home. This does not solve either problem of children's health and behaviour or the health of the planet.

If you want to have an understanding of what lunchbox rubbish looks like, take a look at the image below. As part of The Real Food Lunchbox Project, the school looked at how much waste from lunchbox packets were collected. Every day, 320 students created two washing baskets full of rubbish. This was equated to one small shipping container a year!

2 WASHING BASKETS OF SINGLE-USE RUBBISH COLLECTED EVERY DAY!

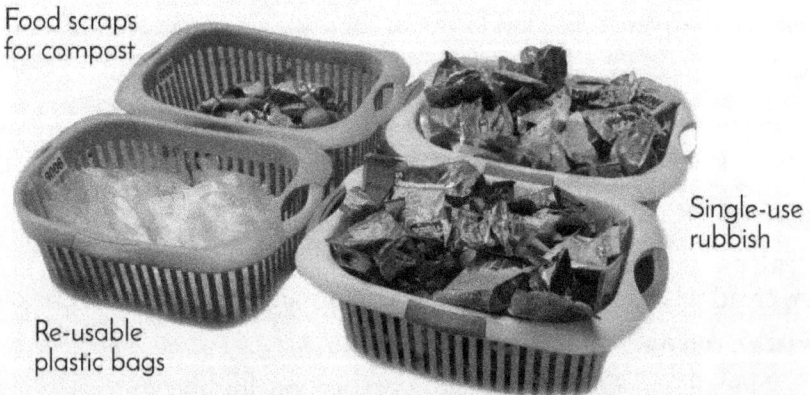

Food scraps for compost

Re-usable plastic bags

Single-use rubbish

In Adelaide, one school teacher worked out that on average, every student produced one zip lock bag a day. This equated to approximately 250,000 zip lock bags a year going into landfill for that one school. Now keeping in mind that our research has found most Australian children are having two processed packet foods in their lunchbox a day, it would mean this one school would be putting 500,000 packets plus 250,000 zip lock bags into landfill.

The Government of South Australia's Wipe Out Waste project run by KESAB Environmental Solutions found that SA schools put on average 950,000 lunchbox packet foods into waste per year. It is estimated the cost of this is approximately $300,000 per year.[46]

If children simply halved the amount of processed packet food they brought to school, imagine how much money schools could save on waste management costs. This money could be diverted back into spending on educational resources or other initiatives to support teacher and student wellbeing.

There are over 9,000 schools across Australia. Can you imagine the amount of waste created every day from what we send our kids to school with to eat? Imagine that for a year. Then for their whole school life. Quite clearly, this is not sustainable for our planet.

Packing real food nourishes our children's body and brain, plus the planet too.

---

5 Simple Actions You Can Take

It would be awesome if we could all take these five simple actions to help reduce lunchbox rubbish, and help make this world a better place for our kids to live in.

1. Talk to your kids about the bigger picture

It's important we get our kids thinking about the bigger picture of the world. Start talking to them about the rubbish we create from the foods we eat. Ask them to think about the amount of rubbish their school would create. The Cool Australia website (**https://www.coolaustralia. org/**) is a fantastic resource you may want to look at with your kids.

They have developed a great waste fact sheet with some pretty scary stats on it about Australia and our waste.

Children also really don't like the idea of hurting animals, so you may also be interested in getting them to have a look around the awesome Ocean Crusaders website (**http://oceancrusaders.org/**). There is lots of great info about what our rubbish is doing to the waterways and the animals that live in it.

2. Make lunchbox food fun and easy to eat

Have conversations about how important lunchbox food is to their growth and development. Ask your kids to help choose what fruit and vegetables and mains they want in their lunchbox for the week. A suggestion is to choose a number of options you are happy with and ask your children to choose from those. The conversation could go something like this – carrots, beans, broccoli and cherry tomatoes are in season this week, which two would you like included in your lunchbox this week. What you are doing here is managing your child's expectation that they will have vegetables in their lunchbox, but you're giving them ownership for which ones they want to have.

Make it fun by including fruits and vegetables of different colours (e.g. cucumber and cherry tomatoes) and cutting food different ways (e.g. sticks and rounds). Be sure to make the food so it's finger food. This way it's easier to eat, more appealing to the eyes and hopefully can get eaten before the playtime bell goes.

If you want help with how to create fun lunchboxes with plenty of finger foods, you may wish to check out
The 5 Minute Healthy Lunchbox System eCourse.

3. Remove at least one packet from your child's lunchbox

If your child is used to having a popper style drink, just tell your children you won't be sending juice to school anymore. Water is all they need. Be sure to explain about those pesky plastic straws and wrappers too. Read the ingredients of the packets you put in lunchboxes and together choose at least one to remove and replace with real food. Slowly, over time, delete the packaged food completely and replace it with homemade creations you and the children have made together. Get Nana or Granny in on this one, I'm sure the grandparents would love to assist.

4. Stop using plastic wrap and plastic bags

Purchase some great reusable zippered bags, and scrap using plastic wrap or zip lock bags. (Refer to appendices at the back of this book for suppliers I trust.)

My suggestion is to talk to your kids about the importance of these bags to help save wildlife, and hence it is important for them to bring the bags home. Then get them to shop online with you to choose their designs and colour. Remember, reusable items are an investment. They will save you money in the long term and help preserve the world our kids are growing up in too.

If you really want to keep buying processed foods, buy bigger packets of them, then break them down into these smaller reusable bags for school. Buying the bigger bags will also save you money. You pay for the convenience of having smaller lunchbox friendly packets.

5. Follow these steps for yourself

Practice what you preach and role model what you want the kids to do. If you think you can buy things, pop them on the top shelf in the pantry and keep them for yourself, then know your kids are likely to see this even if you think they don't. This kind of behaviour sends the message that it's okay to hide food and eat it when no one is watching. If you look at this as an education opportunity, you could buy whatever it is, in full view of the household and enjoy it with the kids, talking about how it's a "sometimes" food.

PART 3:

What do we do now?

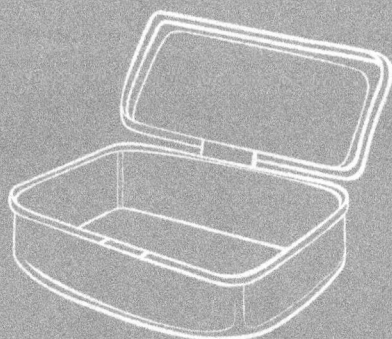

Chapter 10
The Case for a National Food Policy for Schools

Schools are dealing with the melting pot of factors as best they can, including the way students eat and play today and the dynamics going on at home. I do believe initiatives like Breakfast Club, Crunch&Sip®, Munch & Move, or shorter brain breaks early on in the day are valuable. The focus on providing healthy foods from canteens is important too because children are eating junk food most days. They don't need more of it from the canteen. However, the fact remains the foods that are in the school lunchbox are a big issue – this is what most children are eating at school each day.

Many schools are hesitant to tackle the issue of lunchboxes and perhaps others don't realise the significance of the lunchbox. From our own recent surveys of schools who participated in The Mad Food

Science Program, 88% of children still bring their lunchboxes from home.[47] If we consider children have recess and lunch at school, five days a week, then this means about 30-40% of their nutrition for those days is supposed to come from their lunchbox. This nutrition is supposed to fuel the children for the learning and playing hours. It seems absolutely crazy that we don't tackle lunchboxes as an issue.

The Division of Power

At present, both health and education are managed at a state level. This means across Australia, there are a myriad of different approaches to food. Whilst every state has policies in place, the funds and resources to monitor the policies are lacking, therefore the policies are not being enforced. It's a bit like a toothless tiger.

From what we see from visiting schools and from what we hear from teachers who reach out to us, I believe it's time for the Federal Government to take responsibility. I believe **all types** of schools (Government Schools and non-Government) would benefit from a National Food Policy mandated by the Federal Government.

Given the amount of emotion that exists around food, it is understandable why schools are hesitant to tackle lunchbox foods. This is why The Root Cause recommended a National Food Policy for Schools to the Federal Senate Select Committee into the Obesity Epidemic in Australia. Schools need to be supported by the Federal Government so they can powerfully manage the food that comes into the school. In putting forward the recommendation, I suggested these guidelines be consistent across all states, allowing schools to work together sharing how the guidelines are working for them, and how they can be improved.

Model Schools from Other Countries

We should look to what other countries are doing to learn how children are fed at school. In countries such as France, Japan, Norway, and even the UK, the eating breaks are treated as part of the educational journey.

Children are taught life skill such as:
- Manners and respect for those preparing and serving their food
- How to carry their food safely
- To eat and socialise at the same time
- Patience as they wait in line or for everyone to finish
- To clean up after themselves
- And in some schools, to even wash up and wipe down the tables

They tend to have a longer play time too. I witnessed this system in a UK school when I visited in 2018. The system is not perfect. The children have to line up for their food, but the reality is it's teaching them the skill of patience. Each school has a "lunch lady" who has guidelines of what food to cook including recipes, where to shop and how much can be spent. I noticed some recipes use too much sugar, but I believe this will be addressed in the coming years as the UK is tackling the issues around sugar in food thanks to the wonderful campaigning work of Jamie Oliver. On the positive side, the children all ate a hot lunch that had a combination of vegetables, complex carbohydrates and some protein. They sat and enjoyed eating their lunch together, then cleaned up and went out to play.

I sat in and observed the students when they came back to their classroom. They were ready to learn. There was only one child who would be considered "off task" (not doing what the teacher had asked). This child was not being disruptive to the other students or disrespectful to the teacher, she was just looking around. I spoke to one of the teachers about this. She said her belief was because the children had eaten properly, and then had plenty of play time, they understood when they were in the classroom, it was time to learn and get on with the tasks they'd been set.

This is a very different experience to what I have seen and experienced first-hand here in Australian schools. I am seeing children fuelled on high sugar, fat, salt and additive laden foods. It's eaten quickly, followed by a short play period, before returning to the classroom where they are expected to sit and be attentive. It's not working. In many Australian schools you will find many teachers purposefully plan to do activities like art and crafts after lunchbreak because they recognise not a lot of learning happens after lunch.

Leader Schools

If we continue to look a little closer to home, we can find examples of schools who see a noticeable change in children's behaviour and results when their school time eating habits are addressed. Let's have a look at a couple.

A New Zealand School Principal, Susan Dunlop, from Yendarra School was concerned about the behaviour of children in her school. She believed it was connected to the children drinking too many sugary drinks. She said, "There was a culture of fizzy drinks at the school; parents were coming into the school drinking them, as well as children. Behaviour was bad, attendance was bad, truancy was a problem. We had aggressive, overweight children."[48]

Susan implemented a water only policy but made it easy for parents and students. Each student was given a water bottle and new water fountains were installed around the school, so children had easy access to water. Susan makes it clear the water only initiative was not a rule but rather a high expectation for students. There was only one complaint from a parent. The school began seeing results immediately. They observed improvements in behaviour, attendance and learning outcomes. Over time, they saw more substantial results. There was a reduction in waistlines and in dental cavities.

The school used the water only initiative as a catalyst to address healthy food and they even tackled lunchboxes. They began to celebrate healthy food that was brought to school. They took photos of children with healthy lunchboxes and posted them around the school. It became cool to have healthy lunches and more lunches from home started to be healthy with packaged foods being reduced. Parents are supported with information about food choices, food preparation and more. The

Tuckshop was changed to healthy options too. Yendara's success has come by celebrating healthy food.

In Mount Isa Queensland, forward thinking Principal Byron Burke launched a nutrition program at Sunset State School offering all students breakfast, morning tea and lunch, free of charge. The program was originally trialled for Prep students, but was so successful Mr Burke decided to roll it out to the whole school. After two years of running the program, the results were outstanding:

- Improvements in attendance from 78.6% to 91.3%
- Reduction in skin sores
- Children are concentrating for longer
- Relieving pressure on teachers, as the students are ready to learn

---

"From an education perspective as well, these kids are having the right nutrition for their brains, so they're able to focus for longer periods of time."
PREP TEACHER, SARAH MCKENZIE

The school receives no extra funding for this nutrition program but Mr Burke has seen the results and has chosen to prioritise student welfare.[49]

Imagine what could be available to children's health, attendance rates, academic results, and teacher stress if Australian children were all fed nourishing fruits, vegetables and sandwiches as part of a National Food Policy for schools. I find the prospect of this very exciting and I would love to see the Government pilot more schools doing what Mr Burke does.

The School Ecosystem

When I refer to the school ecosystem, I am talking about all the different touch points in the school environment where students receive messages about food. Remember, it is often not what is said but what is seen that sends long lasting messages to children.

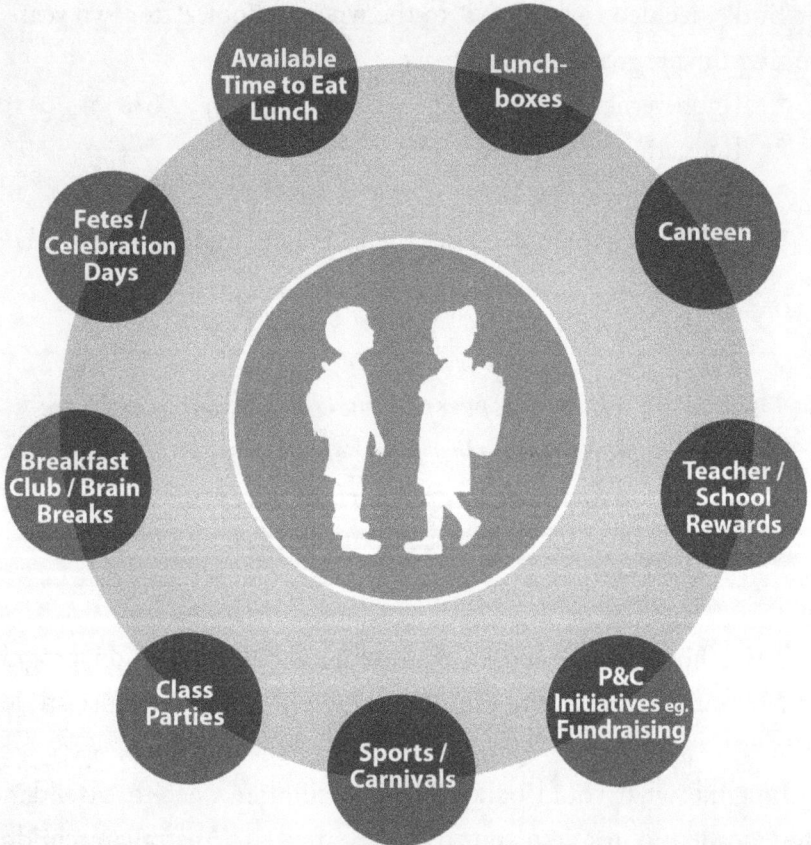

I read a report about using foods as rewards in school and it had this quote. I think it sums up this situation perfectly.

"Rewarding children with unhealthy foods in school undermines our efforts to teach them about good nutrition. It's like teaching children a lesson on the importance of not smoking, and then handing out ashtrays and lighters to the kids who did the best job listening."

MARLENE SCHWARTZ, PH.D., DEPUTY DIRECTOR, RUDD CENTRE FOR
FOOD POLICY AND OBESITY, YALE UNIVERSITY

Now let's relate this back to the school ecosystem. We know children need physical activity. It's an important part of the curriculum. Schools host sports carnivals which support the curriculum and to encourage physical activity. At the same event or on another occasion they then sell lollies, chips, soft drinks afterwards to raise money. All the great work for their health by way of the physical activity is totally undone by the rubbish children eat afterwards. At many schools, children are allowed to be spectators rather than participants, and these children who aren't even exercising, are buying the rubbish too. What's the message children are getting? Do or don't do some exercise and reward yourself with sweets. That's just one example of mixed messages.

We know 94% of children are not eating enough fruits and vegetables[50] and they are eating excessive amounts processed food every day[51]. We need actions that will change this dynamic in the school system. Actions that take the implementation and financial cost away from the schools allowing them to focus on the important role of education.

My Hope for a National Food Policy for Schools

I strongly believe to curb and reverse the issues we are seeing in Children's Health; the Federal Government need to create a National Food Policy for Schools and at the very least:

- Set a water only policy for schools.
- Provide each school with money for fruit and vegetables for each student. The funds should be enough to feed children a piece of fruit per day and at least one serve of vegetables a day, along with say a dip or smoothie, plus the resources to prepare the produce.
- That children be provided with real food as snacks at school from this fund every day.
- Provide funding to support schools to have facilities (e.g. fridges and ovens) to allow them to prepare and serve real food.
- Encourage parents to focus on providing a nourishing main lunch and provide them with simple instructions on what foods are best. Ultimately, it would be great if the Government could fund lunches – at least a great sandwich, as well as fruits and vegetables – for every student.
- Mandate a list of "blacklisted" foods for schools, such as the flavoured chips, crackers and muesli bars that have additives that may potentially affect learning and behaviour.
- Food sent to school should be "nude" – no packaging. (See the the chapter on Environmental Impacts).
- A return of cooking classes (historically Home Economics) as part of the curriculum.
- A basic food garden to help educate children about where food comes from.

While this may sound radical, The Real Food Lunchbox Project we worked on with a whole school demonstrated when fruit and vegetables are provided, and they are the norm for what kids eat, the kids will happily eat fruits and vegetables. We should not underestimate the power of kids just wanting to fit in. It's the reason why kids who have healthy lunchboxes are always complaining to their parents about why it's not fair that they don't have chips, biscuits etc. Because they feel not normal. We need to normalise fruits and vegetables. It should also be recognised if kids (and even adults) are given a choice – healthy food put alongside packaged processed food (made with food and marketing science to send exciting messages to our brains), most will choose the processed food. Offering only the healthy options means that's what gets eaten. That's what's normal.

Through the use of buying power of produce, in the Real Food Lunchbox Project, we were able to source produce for fruit and a serve of vegetables, for just seventy-five cents a day. This was negotiated between the school and the local Farmers Markets. The school used their own resources within the school to prepare the produce each day. In overseas countries where schools provide food, the councils provide schools with funds for the food and also to cover the cost of a "lunch lady".

A fund provided by the government also takes away the common parental complaints fruits and vegetables are too expensive, or they don't have time to pack them. It is also likely to mean children who are from food insecure homes get the much needed nourishment they miss out on normally.

If we want to improve children's health and academic performance, then we have to spend money addressing the problem schools are facing. The reality is schools are a business. They are in the business of helping children reach their full potential so they can go on and contribute to this country.

In any business, when something is not working, employees and management look at what's not working, and they take action to fix it. In schools that recognise food is a problem, if they try to address it with parents, they often are met with a backlash or the school receives flack for lunchbox shaming, or worse, the media makes a light-hearted story out of it.

Just recently a morning TV show aired a segment about an NSW school banning parents from having fast food like KFC and McDonalds delivered to schools for lunch. The TV show turned it into a big laugh fest about one of the commentator's heritage and how his lunch used to be different when he was at school. There was no recognition for the school and their efforts to prevent childhood illness.

So how can a school run an effective business – and help this generation of children fulfil their potential – if their hands are tied because of the response from parents and the media?

This needs to stop. We need to recognise schools are on the receiving end of school lunchbox food and they need to be able to take action. A National Food Policy for Schools would provide them with the necessary support to be able to take action.

It is my belief the answer lies with the Federal Government. The Federal Government has the power to mandate change if they develop a strategy to tackle and fund food in schools. The strategy needs to address all food touch points in schools and the funding, as a minimum, should support water only policies and fruit and vegetables for every student and teacher.

The Root Cause will continue to advocate for real food in schools at a National and State Level. We'd love to hear your thoughts on what action you would like to see the Government take to support parents and schools to have a real food policy. The best way to share your thoughts is to email **belinda@therootcause.com.au** with the subject line – Real Food Advocate.

Chapter 11
A Simple Way to Read Packet Labels

There is nothing wrong with having processed packet foods in your pantry or fridge. All the contributors to this book have some in theirs. But, with so much choice at the supermarket it is now an **essential life skill** to be able to read a packet label. It is imperative these life skills are taught to our children too. Processed packet foods are not going away. They are firmly entrenched as part of the way most Australians eat.

Whatever you buy at the shops and bring home will be eaten. Buy and bring home foods you have consciously chosen.

One of the best ways you can take care of your child's health (and your own), is to start being more conscious of the sorts of packet foods you buy. Read the ingredients list. Ask yourself:

1. Will this food help my body or not help my body?
2. Do I really want to be putting this in my body, or my family's bodies?
3. Can I find a better alternative, either on the shelf or from a recipe?

Parents often tell us they don't have time for this. That's why we've written this book. To give you a helping hand to get started with the most common lunchbox packet foods. However, we do strongly recommend you take the time to learn the simple steps in this chapter in how to read packet labels. Get your children involved. By doing so, you will ultimately get to the point where your children are saying no, they don't want the food for their one body for life. Reading packet labels and becoming food literate is a life skill they will need now but more importantly, for when they leave your nest.

Overview of Food Labels

Although Francine Bell covered this in a great amount of detail in her chapters earlier in the book, this serves as a quick re-cap.

Labelling laws require ingredients to be listed, but if an ingredient is made up of two or more ingredients (these are called compound ingredients), and one of the compound ingredients makes up less than 5% of the end food, it doesn't have to be noted as an ingredient unless it is an allergen.

Catch-all ingredients like "spices" and "flavours" disguise what the ingredients really are. Spices and flavours can include additives that have similar effects as MSG, but these do not have to be disclosed if they make up less than 5% of the spices or flavours. It's interesting to note, companies are not required to disclose what makes up their flavours because this is considered to be intellectual property, and someone may copy it. A bit like KFC's secret herbs and spices.

"Flavours" can be made of many ingredients - 50, 100, 200 - seriously we just don't know. Natural flavours, which to many sound perfectly fine and harmless, just means they have been derived from using plant, spices, or herbs. Be aware "both artificial and natural flavours are made by "flavourists" in a laboratory by blending either "natural" chemicals or "synthetic" chemicals to create flavourings."[52]

Look out for the words "No Added Sugar" or "No Added MSG". This means the manufacturer has not added them, but it may well be that it's added in some other form. A classic example of this are beverages sweetened with likes of aspartame.

Additives can be naturally occurring substances (salt, sugar, vinegar etc.) but many are now chemically produced, offering no nutritional value. Many are specifically designed by food scientists to get us wanting to eat more of their product. Let's be 100% clear about this. Food manufacturers are using food science to engineer foods to make them irresistible, so we want to keep eating more and more of them.[53]

In Australia, there are currently over 300 additives and preservatives approved by FSANZ, and each have been given what's called an INS number. They can be broken down into the following groups:

INS Number	Description
100-199	Colours
200-299	Preservatives and Acidity regulators
300-399	Antioxidants, Acidity regulators, Stabilisers, Anti Caking Agents
400-499	Emulsifiers, Humectants, Vegetable Gums,
500-599	Anti-caking Agents, Firming Agents, Stabilisers, Gelling Agents, Acidity Regulators
600-899	Flavour Enhancers
900-1202	Glazing agents, Sweeteners, Bleaching agents, Propellants and Gases, Antifoaming agents, Emulsifiers
1400-1450	Modified Starches (Thickeners, Stabilisers and Binders)
1503-1521	Humectants, Antifoaming agents, Dispersing agents

Before delving into the simple steps of reading a label, let's just have a look at the three main areas of a packet:

1. **The Front** – this is where you will find the name of the product and the marketing messages the food manufacturer wants you to see. Things like: "30% Less Sugar", "No Artificial Colours or Flavours", "Gluten Free", "Lunchbox Friendly", "Canteen Approved" and the list goes on.
2. **The Back – Nutrition Information Panel** (the box with all the numbers). This is hugely important because it contains information on the average amount of energy, protein, fat,

saturated fat, carbohydrates, sugars and sodium in the food. However, a simpler way to work out "What's In My Food?" is to look at the ingredients list.

3. **The Back – Ingredients.** The Ingredients are usually located underneath or to the left or right of the Nutritional Information Panel. You may need to hunt for them as they are often in small print. Looking at the ingredients is the simplest way to answer, "What's In My Food?" In doing the product reviews for this book, we have noticed some manufacturers have dropped the word "Ingredients" and use words like "Contains", or they even just list the ingredients with no title.

Note: You may also see marketing messages on the back of the packet.

The Five Simple Steps to Read a Packet Label

There are five simple steps to reading packet labels. You can have fun teaching your kids this too. This method may be slightly different as traditionally taught by others but this is the method we have found makes it super simple for kids to understand. If you've read Chapter 4 about the foods your kids need to thrive, hopefully you have had a chance to talk to your children about why the food they eat is so important. This should make it a bit easier to get your children involved in reading packet labels.

1. **Ignore the front of the packet.** Turn the packet around and find the word "ingredients".
2. **Count the number of ingredients.** If you find more than 6 ingredients, consider putting that product back on the shelf.
3. **Look for "Sugar", "Salt" or "Fat" in the Ingredients.** If you see the words "sugar", "salt" or "fat" listed in first 3 ingredients, consider putting that product back on the shelf.

4. **Count how many teaspoons of sugar per serve.** This requires doing a little maths with the numbers in the Nutritional Information Panel. Remember 1 teaspoon = 4.2 grams – to make it easy for your kids and yourself, round down to 4 and use your 4 times tables.

5. **Look up the additives to learn their POTENTIAL effects.** If the packet contains additives, preservatives, colours, etc, look up the number or name in "The Chemical Maze" app or a similar resource to answer, "What's In My Food?"

These steps are sequential. Step 1 applies to ALL products. If your product passes Step 2, move on to Step 3, and so on. At each step, make a conscious choice about whether it is wise to proceed onto the next step, or if would it be better to put the packet back on the shelf and find a better one.

You may even prefer to work out how you can make an equivalent at home. We live in a blessed world with the internet because at our fingertips. You can easily find a recipe for almost every food you would normally buy from the supermarket. When you make it at home, you know exactly what ingredients have gone in it.

In the next section, I've gone into more detail on each of the steps:

Step 1 – Ignore the Front of the Packet, Turn It Over and Find the Ingredients.

The front of the packet is purely marketing. A marketer's job is to find the right combination of colours, pictures and words that get you to buy the product. And you know what? You are their secret weapon. They rely on busy parents being unconscious consumers.

They rely on this busyness to get you to turn a blind eye to what you know you should be feeding your kids (i.e. not their products), so everything on the front of the packet is designed to make you feel better about turning a blind eye. Companies spend huge amounts of money on marketing, and it's all designed to make you feel comfortable with the purchase. Every aspect is considered—the colours on the packet, the shape of the packaging, the words used, the images used, the type, font, angles of wording, the sound of the packaging when you touch the packet and of course, where it sits on the supermarket shelf. Scientists in laboratories are also paid big money to be responsible for the actual taste of the product. Everything is designed to get you to buy this product, regardless of whether or not it is nutritious for our body.

In the example above, I ask kids to ignore the picture of the sports person clearly leaping up to grab the ball. I'm asking you to ignore the words, "Energy Dairy Snack, Calcium, Iron, B Vitamins & Minerals". Also ignore "Available for On The Go". That's all marketing. Turn the packet over. Take a look at the Ingredients List. This is the quickest way of knowing "What's In My Food?"

The ingredients list is usually located just below or to the left or right of the Nutrition Information Panel (the box with all the numbers). For the purposes of the book, I have separated out the ingredients from the Nutrition Information Panel in this photo, however, on the actual packaging, the ingredients are to the left of the information panel.

Here's what you need to think about:
- The ingredients are listed in order of weight from the largest quantity used to the smallest quantity in the food.
- Be wary if the first ingredient does not match what the product is supposed to be. For instance, if you are looking at fruit juice, and something other than fruit is shown first, then leave this product behind.
- Be especially wary when sugar is listed as the first ingredient. Personally, if sugar was the first ingredient, I'd leave this product behind too.
- Be alert for ingredients which you know are not good for you, ingredients that have long, chemical-sounding names, or ingredients you can't identify.
- Look out for ingredients that appear multiple times but under different names. For example, trans fats (which are the worst possible fats for you) often get listed as partially hydrogenated oil or hydrogenated oil. Sugar can also show up in many different names. (See list in appendix).

Step 2 – Count the Number of Ingredients
If the ingredients list has more than 6 ingredients, it's usually a sign the product has been, at best moderately processed, and is unlikely to offer much to help our one body for life. If there is more than six, you may wish to consider putting it back on the shelf and searching for a better choice.

The ingredients listed can often contain words that are just plain confusing and impossible for the average person to get their tongue around. The easiest way to count the ingredients is just to count the commas. Everywhere there is a comma, it is a new ingredient. Add on the last ingredient before the full stop.

Sometimes you will see an ingredient listed then it will have brackets next to it with more ingredients inside the brackets. This means the ingredients inside the brackets are used to make the ingredient in front of the bracket. If you see this, count the commas (ingredients) inside the brackets too. Let's do an example here:

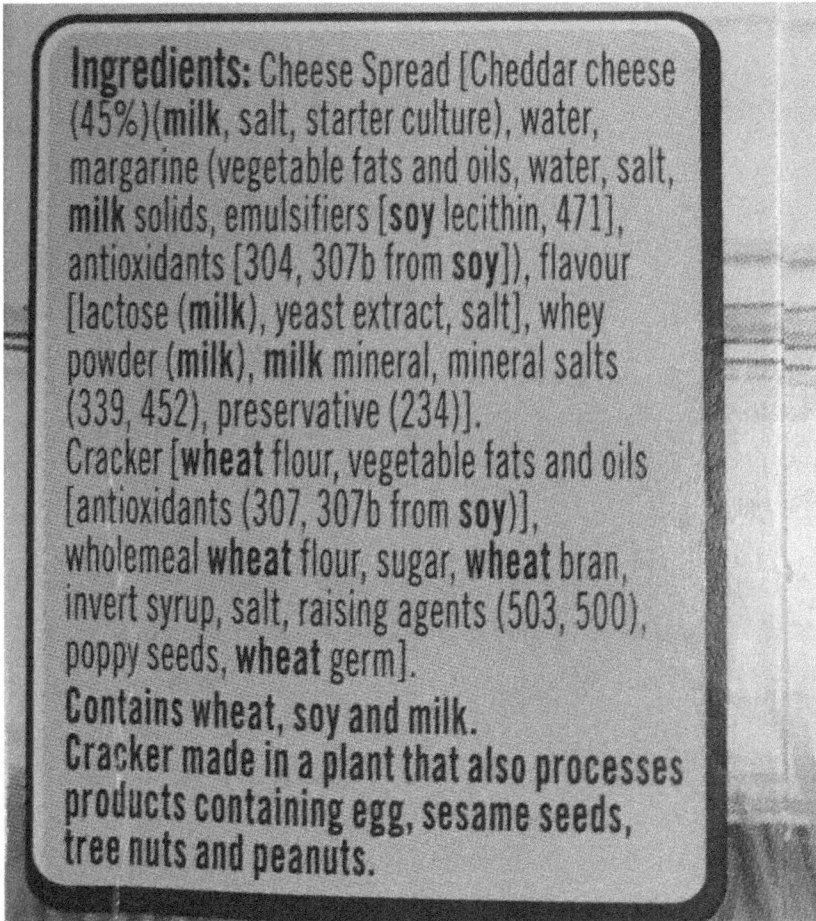

Ingredients: Cheese Spread [Cheddar cheese (45%)(milk, salt, starter culture), water, margarine (vegetable fats and oils, water, salt, milk solids, emulsifiers [soy lecithin, 471], antioxidants [304, 307b from soy]), flavour [lactose (milk), yeast extract, salt], whey powder (milk), milk mineral, mineral salts (339, 452), preservative (234)].
Cracker [wheat flour, vegetable fats and oils [antioxidants (307, 307b from soy)], wholemeal wheat flour, sugar, wheat bran, invert syrup, salt, raising agents (503, 500), poppy seeds, wheat germ].
Contains wheat, soy and milk.
Cracker made in a plant that also processes products containing egg, sesame seeds, tree nuts and peanuts.

In this example, there are 2 sets of ingredients – one for the cheese spread, and one for the crackers. We'll count the ingredients of the cheese spread below. For ease of counting, we have separated the list into lines, bolded the commas and added an extra space, so they are easy for you to see.

Ingredient	Count
Cheddar cheese (milk, salt, starter culture),	3
water,	1
margarine (vegetable fats and oils, water, salt, milk solids, emulsifiers [soy lecithin, 471], antioxidants [304, 307b from soy]) ,	8
flavour [lactose (milk), yeast extract, salt],	3
whey powder (milk),	1
milk mineral,	1
mineral salts (339, 452),	2
preservative (234).	1
Total	**20**

The Cheese Spread is made up of twenty "ingredients". Just as a side note, you can make this cheese spread very easily at home with just 100g of tasty cheese (grate it from the block) and 150g of full fat sour cream. When I asked, "What's In My Food?" for the cheese and the sour cream, I counted seven ingredients all up. Head to the FREE Bonuses to watch me making the cheese spread at home.

Grab your FREE Bonuses for The Lunchbox Effect:
http://thelunchboxeffect.com/bonuses

Step 3 – Look for Sugar, Salt or Fat In the Ingredients?

It is a labelling requirement in Australia that ingredients must be listed in order by weight from the largest to the smallest quantity in the food. This means first three ingredients will make up most of what's in the food.

If sugar, salt and fat are in the first three, then it's likely there may be more than what is healthy for your body or that when you add it to the other processed foods you eat in the day, you may exceed the limits healthy for your body. It is recommended you put these packets back on the shelf. Here's why:

Sugar

Broadly speaking, sugar falls into two categories.

1. **Natural sugar.** This occurs in whole pieces of fruit and vegetables and dairy based products. Natural sugar does not need to be listed as an ingredient and in its whole state is not harmful to the body because it is bound up with fibre, which slows the release of sugar in the body's blood stream.
2. **Free or Added Sugar.** This is processed sugar and is added as an ingredient in processing. This does need to be listed as an ingredient.

If you see sugar as an ingredient, then it means the product contains free (added) sugar. It is this form of sugar we need to concern ourselves most with from a health perspective. Unlike fruit and vegetables that have all important fibre to slow down the use of sugar, free or added sugar does not have that. What is even more tricky is in Australia, sugar can show up as an ingredient using over 60 different names[54] (See the appendix for these names).

A general rule of thumb is if a product contains added sugar, aim for 5g or less of sugar per 100g.
That Sugar Movement (https://thatsugarmovement.com/how-much-sugar-should-i-eat/)[55]

Free/Added Sugar Recommendations

The World Health Organisation (WHO) recommends for optimal health we should be limiting our free sugars to 5% of our total energy intake. In Australia, we tend to use the term added sugar rather than free sugars, but free sugar is a bit broader because it not just includes the sugars added by the manufacturer, but also the "sugars that are naturally present in honey, syrups and fruit juices."[56]

The natural sugar in fruits and vegetables is bound with natural fibre, which makes all the difference to the way it is metabolised in the body. Another sugar not included as "free sugar" is the natural sugars present in milk, i.e. lactose.

The World Health Organisation recommendation states that adults can safely consume the equivalent of approximately six teaspoons of "added" sugar per day. It's important to note that this is a recommendation across *all* the foods eaten in a day. In Australia, a teaspoon is 4g, so the recommendation is 24g of "free sugar" is a safe allowance for adults per day.

It is an interesting and eye-opening exercise to keep track of the number of teaspoons of added sugar you consume over a 24 hour period.

Sugar Recommendations for Children

As children grow, their energy requirements change. This can be due to their growth stage, gender and the amount of physical activity they do. The upper limit for sugar intake can vary from 3 to 6 teaspoons a day.[57]

It is important to note, it is advised children under two should not be consuming added sugar at all. Yet, for many children, the foods they are eating at this age contain added sugar. It is in these early years that children's palates and reward centres in the brain are being bombarded with sugar, so the taste of sugar becomes what they "need" when they taste food.

For most primary aged children, the upper limit for added sugar is 3-5 teaspoons (again depending on their age and level of physical activity). Let's summarise and have a look at what's currently happening in Australia when it comes to the amount of added sugar we are eating per day.

Age	Recommendations per day[58]	Current Australian Consumption per day[59]
Adults	6 tsp / 24g of sugar	~16 tsp / 65g of sugar (19-30yo)
Children < 2	No added sugar	Not reported on
Children 2-3	~2 tsp / ~8g of sugar	8 tsp / 32g of sugar
Children 4-8	3-5 tsp / 12-20g of sugar	12 tsp / 48g of sugar
Children 9-13	3-5 tsp / 12-20g of sugar	16 tsp / 64g of sugar
Children 14-18	4-5 tsp / 16-20g of sugar	~18 tsp / 73g of sugar

As you can see from this table, all age groups reported on are eating significantly more added sugar than WHO recommendations. This over consumption is concerning but the picture for long-term health becomes even more disturbing when you combine it with the fact that many children (and adults) are participating in less physical activity these days.

What's also alarming is a whopping 46% of young adults aged 18-24 are now overweight or obese.[60] This does not start at this age; it creeps in over years of consuming poor quality foods.

Sodium (Salt)

If salt is added to a product, it will be listed as an ingredient, but it's displayed in the nutritional information panel as sodium. This requires you to do a mathematical conversion to work out how many grams of salt there are before you can compare it to the recommendations for salt. It's just much easier to remember if it's in the top three ingredients, when you add it to everything else you have in the day, it may take you over the salt recommendations for your body.

Salt Recommendation

The World Health Organization recommends a maximum salt intake of 5 g/day (a little over a teaspoon), yet it is reported Australia's salt intake is twice this recommended level.[61]

If you want to make a conscious effort to calculate the amount of salt per packet of what you are eating, Catherine Saxelby's Food Watch website has a great easy **Quick Sodium and Salt Converter Table**. Or using the nutritional information panel, you can work out if the product is low, medium or high in salt. Follow Catherine's simple guidelines outlined below[62]:

- Low salt products are less than 120mg sodium per 100g
- Medium salt products over 120mg but less than 600mg sodium per 100g
- High salt products are more than 600mg per 100g
- Aim for 2000 mg of sodium (5g salt / 1 teaspoon) per day. This is across all foods.

The table below shows the contrast between current recommendations and consumption rates for primary aged children.[63]

Age	National Health & Medical Research Council's Recommendations	Australian Heath Survey Data
4-8 yo	Upper limit 3.5g per day	5.1g per day
9-13 yo	Upper limit 5g per day	6.2g per day

Like sugar, you can see we are consuming way too much salt than what's recommended. Too much sodium in what we eat can contribute to health conditions such as high blood pressure, stroke, and increases the risk of heart disease. One important way you can counterbalance salt intake is by increasing the intake of potassium through eating more fruits and vegetables. Unfortunately, as we know in Australia, only 6% of children are eating the recommended amounts of fruits and vegetables per day. Therefore, our kids are eating too much salt and not enough vegetables. Can you see the long-term risk here?

The George Institute has specifically identified lunchbox packet foods as a way to lower the salt intake by children[64]. You can get help with lowering salt levels by using their FoodSwitch app.

"We've shown that children can avoid consuming almost 4g of salt if parents make the right choices for their lunchboxes."
DR JACQUI WEBSTER, THE GEORGE INSTITUTE.

Fat

In Chapter 4, Jo Atkinson shared about the important role "good" fats play for our body and brain. These fats generally come from wholefood sources (e.g. avocado, eggs, olive oil, real butter etc). Most fats (including oils) used by food manufacturers in lunchbox packet foods do not fall into the good fats variety. They are cheaper and nastier for our body and brain. These are the fats, when eaten in excess, lead to inflammation in our body and contribute to long-term health conditions such as heart disease, diabetes type 2, auto immune conditions and more.

The World Health Organisation recommends we limit our total fats to 30% of our total energy intake per day and saturations fats to 10% of total energy intake and trans-fats to 1% of total energy intake.[65]

This recommendation makes it much more difficult for us to assess how much fat we're consuming which is why I recommend that when it comes to lunchbox packet foods, if fat is in the top three, then put it back.

Too much added sugar, too much sodium and too much saturated and trans-fat have all been identified as risks to our health. Statistics show us children are consuming way more than the recommended amounts in all three of these areas. This must change. The long-term health of Australian children is at risk here.

Added sugar, extra sodium, saturated fats and trans-fats are found predominantly in discretionary foods. For the sake of the health of Australian kids, we need to move away from eating so many discretionary foods and be smart about the ones we allow our children to have. It's important to be vigilant when choosing your discretionary food. Read the ingredients list with every choice and when sugar, sodium, fat or oils appear in the first 3 ingredients choose again.

There is a simplicity to eating real wholefoods –
Choose food as close as possible to its original source.
The closer it is to it's original source, the more likely it is to
help our one body for life.

Step 4 – Count How Many Teaspoons of Sugar per Serve

Just to reiterate, The World Health Organisation free or added sugar recommendation across ALL foods and drinks eaten across the whole day (breakfast, lunch, snacks, dinner, dessert) is:

- Adults, maximum 6 teaspoons (24g) for the whole day
- Children under 2, nil
- Children 2-3yo, approx. 2 tspns (8g)
- Children 4-8yo, 3-5 tspsns (12-20g) depending on age and activity level
- Children 9-13yo, 3-5 tspsns (12-20g) depending on age and activity level
- Older children – 3-6 tspns (12-24g) depending on age and activity level

To work out how much sugar there is in what you're about to eat, you need to look at the Nutritional Information Panel. This can get a little tricky because the Nutritional Information Panel only lists the total sugars (natural + added) in a product. This makes it difficult for us consumers to truly know how much added sugar is in a product. One of the recommendations from the Federal Senate Select Committee from August 2018 was to list our added sugars separately but at the time of publishing, this recommendation has not been enacted.

Notwithstanding this, it is usually a pretty good indicator of added sugar if:

- If you see sugar (or one of the many names for it) in the top three ingredients - then you know it's a major ingredient in the overall formulation of the product.
- If you count the number of times sugar in its different names shows up in the ingredients list. It's likely when you add up all the amounts from those different names, sugar would be a large part of the ingredients.

Using two examples, we're going to work out the total sugar, and make a judgement call. (Note: I say this because it is your call about whether you want to have this product for your family on whether it has too much sugar.)

When making a judgement call, it is recommended you consider what else your child will be consuming in the day they eat or drink this product. Remembering WHO's recommendations are across all meals and snacks in the day. Therefore, you need to consider the food that will be eaten across the day, not just this one packet. Think about the amount of sugar they will have in their breakfast, snacks, lunch, evening meal, or any dessert. It is very easy for the amount of sugar being eaten to add up way past the recommendations when consuming packet foods.

To work out the sugar, we need to look at serving size, number of serves in the packet and the amount of sugar in the serving you will eat.

Example 1: - Arnott's Tiny Teddies Honey Biscuit

HONEY
BISCUITS
Wheat Flour, Sugar, Vegetable Oil (Contains **Soy**), Honey (5%), Butter (Cream (From **Milk**), Salt), Vegetable Fibre, Salt, Emulsifier (**Soy** Lecithin), Baking Powder, Natural Flavour.
CONTAINS GLUTEN CONTAINING CEREALS, MILK AND SOY.
MAY CONTAIN TRACES OF EGG, PEANUT, SESAME AND TREE NUT.

CHOCOLAT
BISCUITS
Wheat Flou
Powder, Hon
Baking Powc
CONTAINS
MAY CONT

NUTRITION INFORMATION

	QUANTITY PER SERVING	%DAILY INTAKE * (PER SERVING)	QUANTITY PER 100 g	
SERVINGS PER PACKAGE: 5	SERVING SIZE: 25 g			SERVINGS PE
ENERGY	463 kJ	5.3%	1,850 kJ	ENERGY
PROTEIN	1.6 g	3.1%	6.3 g	PROTEIN
FAT, TOTAL	3.3 g	4.7%	13.3 g	FAT, TOTAL
-SATURATED	1.8 g	7.4%	7.1 g	-SATURAT
CARBOHYDRATE	17.9 g	5.8%	71.7 g	CARBOHYDRA
-SUGARS	6.3 g	7.0%	25.2 g	-SUGARS
DIETARY FIBRE	1.2 g	4.0%	4.7 g	DIETARY FIBR
SODIUM	79 mg	3.4%	317 mg	SODIUM

* BASED ON AN AVERAGE ADULT DIET OF 8700 K.I. ALL VALUES CONSIDERED AVERAGES UNLESS OTHERWISE

1. It shows the serving size is 25g, and there are 5 servings in the package. This means there are five packets of 25g in this multi-pack box. Each bag of biscuits is 25g.
2. Scroll down the per serving column (i.e. one packet) to the word sugar. It shows 6.3g of total sugar.
3. Given Tiny Teddy's are marketing towards younger children, this one bag has over half of the amount of sugar recommended for this age group.

To consider how much of this total sugar is added sugar, go back to the ingredients and see where sugar sits. You will see sugar is the second ingredient. This means sugar is a major ingredient in this product. Given this is the case, it's reasonable to expect most of the 1.6 teaspoons of sugar in this bag will be added sugar. This means for the average child doing the average amount of physical activity in a day, this one bag contains over half the amount of recommended added sugar for the entire day across all foods and drinks.

Now it's time for you to make a judgement call about whether you want your child to have this product and if so, how often. Remember to consider what else they eat in the day.

Example 2: - Golden Circle Sunshine Punch 250ml

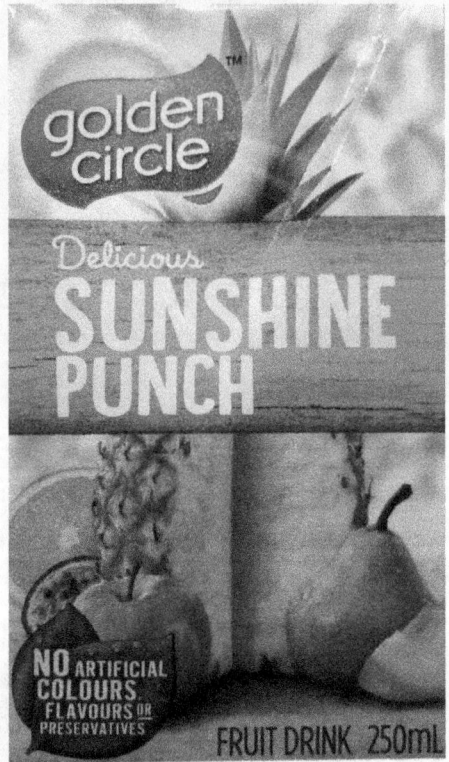

1. It shows the serving size is 250ml, and there is one serving in the package.
2. Scroll down the per serving column to the word sugar. It shows 24.8g of total sugar.
3. This means this Golden Circle Sunshine Punch 250ml juice box contains 6.2 teaspoons of total sugar.

Many people will say, "Oh, it's fruit so most of that will be natural sugars." But it's no longer part of the whole fruit which means the all-important fibre from the whole fruit that slows down the use of the sugar has been removed. Your child's body just sees this as sugar. As per WHO definitions, sugar in juices like this are considered free sugars, and as such, this one juice box has an adult full day serving size of free sugar.

Turning our attention to the ingredients, let's see what else they can tell us,

The ingredients are listed as follows:
- **Water** is the first and main ingredient
- **Reconstituted juice** (25% and lists the different varieties of fruit). Reconstituted means it was fruit that has been squeezed, then the juice is subjected to high heat to remove nearly all the water from it. So essentially it's just the sugars of the fruit without the important fibre that slows down the use of the natural sugars. It's also questionable about the nutrient content that remains following the heat process.
- **Sugar** is the third ingredient. This means sugar is a significant part of this product.
- **Food acids** usually used for preserving.
- **Vitamin C**. Given fruit tends to naturally contain vitamin C, the fact it is being added back in, what does it tell you about the initial processing of the fruit? Also, it is likely this is synthetically made as natural Vitamin C comes from the whole food which has been severely altered in processing this fruit into reconstituted juice.
- **Natural Flavours.** This is a question I always ask kids. Hands up who likes apples or oranges? Who thinks they are tasty? Then why do you think they need to add flavours into this juice? Again, what does this ingredient tell you about

the initial processing of the fruit? Maybe the processes to reconstitute takes away the natural flavours of the fruit. We don't even know what is in this ingredient natural flavours.

- **Stabiliser (Pectin).** It is likely this ingredient is included to help keep the reconstituted juice and water mixed.

So, as well as having the sugar that's been extracted from the fruit initially, it also has additional sugar added into it. A question I love to ask children is whether they think fruit is tasty and sweet. The majority say yes. I then ask them why they think food manufacturers need to add in Natural Flavours to the juice then. Have a think about it. Why do you think they need to add flavours to fruit which is already?

From our travels around Australia, and the survey we conducted of the children in our community, juices are a popular addition to a school lunchbox. The fact there are so many of these on the supermarket shelf (over fifty varieties across three supermarket chains) is also testament to how popular these juices are. Remembering sugar spikes cause an energy spike, then an energy slump, then triggers our body to need another spike. This is exactly what these drinks are doing every school day to kids. Teachers we have spoken to share their experiences of kids who come back to class dosed up on sugar. They mentioned the impact it has on the classroom, the heightened activity from the energy, then the slump because they can no longer concentrate.

Can you imagine being a teacher with a few kids in each class who has to try to encourage learning while children's bodies are dealing with this up and down?

Now I am going to say something which may make me unpopular, but I am going to say it for our teachers and for our kids:

*Please keep juices for home. Do not send them to school.
The best drink for your child at school is water. Water
hydrates and supports your child's body and brain. It will
not cause highs and lows.*

Step 5 – Look Up the Additives to Learn Their Potential Effects

In the beginning of food manufacture, the intention of additives were honourable. They were meant to do good things for people, like to prolong shelf life a little. This was important, especially during war times. Or to preserve foods when nature provided them in abundance during their growing season. But today, I personally believe many additives are food science gone mad. They are added to products for profit, rather than with us consumers and our health in mind.

There has been so much research into additives and preservatives that show some people are affected by them. The effects can be wide and varied—behaviour problems, eczema, dermatitis, asthma, hyperactivity, irritability, sleep disturbances, depression, learning difficulties, coughing, sneezing, nose bleeds, head banging, aggressive behaviour and more. The affects are cumulative, meaning repetitive intake from processed foods causes a build-up in the body's system. and the consequences/ affects are prolonged for the child/ person affected

Sometimes, the effects are cumulative, meaning the additive may not affect the person until they've been eating it a while and it's built up in their system. Sometimes, the affects can be immediate, showing up straight away or within minutes. They can be delayed; showing up an hour, three hours, a day, even three weeks later – it is really hard to pinpoint the problem when symptoms show up so late, suffice to say, the additives and preservatives require investigation every time you consider purchasing processed foods.

Be an advocate for your family's health, become the ingredients' detective. The only way you know if your child is affected by additives is to try removing them from the way you eat for a week or two and see.

The easiest way to look out for additives on a packet label is to look for ingredients that are listed as numbers. It is recommended you use resources such as The Chemical Maze App, Additive Alert App or Fedup.com.au **https://www.fedup.com.au/** to learn more about these ingredients. Francine from Additive Free Kids advises there are also new ingredients that are being used as additives that technically are not additives as defined by FSANZ. Sadly, even if you ring the company, there is no guarantee you will find out what the ingredients are. Do the best you can by looking at the numbers, but also keep playing detective and looking out for any unusual behaviours and sleep patterns in your children.

Once you have looked at the numbers, turn your attention to the name of ingredients you can't pronounce or sound like something you couldn't have in your own pantry. Use the above mentioned resources or the internet to learn more about these.

Look, I know this sounds like a lot of work, but isn't your children's health worth it? It's not like you have to do it every shop, just look at the products you usually buy. Start with the ones you have the most.

You should also be aware food manufacturers know consumers are getting wise and looking out for numbers and strange sounding ingredients, so some are giving ingredients made in the chemistry lab pleasant sounding names. If you see an ingredient and it sounds pleasant, ask yourself if it is an ingredient you could buy off the shelf and add to your food yourself. If you can't, then know it's an ingredient made specifically for large scale food manufacture and is likely to be an additive.

Let's take a look two examples here:

Example 1: - Blue Bolt Gatorade 600ml

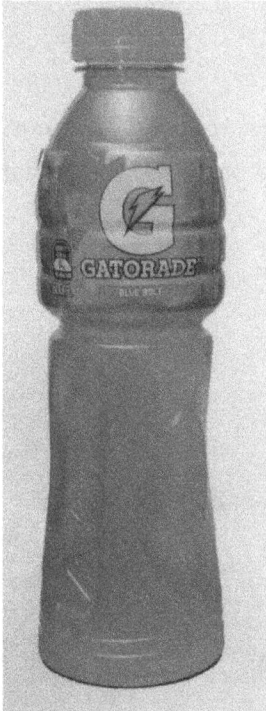

SHAKE WELL REFRIGERATE AFTER OPENING			
NUTRITION INFORMATION			
SERVINGS PER PACK: 1 SERVING SIZE: 600mL			
	AVE QTY PER SERVING	% DAILY INTAKE^ PER SERVING	AVE QTY PER 100mL
ENERGY	618 kJ	7%	103 kJ
PROTEIN	0 g	0%	0 g
FAT, TOTAL	0 g	0%	0 g
- SATURATED	0 g	0%	0 g
CARBOHYDRATE	36 g	12%	6 g
- SUGARS	36 g	40%	6 g
- SUCROSE	33 g		5.5 g
- GLUCOSE	3 g		0.5 g
DIETARY FIBRE, TOTAL	0 g	0%	0 g
SODIUM	306 mg (13.7 mmol)	12%	51 mg (2.3 mmol)
POTASSIUM	135 mg (3.6 mmol)		22.5 mg (0.6 mmol)

^Percentage daily intakes are based on an average adult diet of 8700kJ. Your daily intakes may be higher or lower depending on your energy needs.

STORE IN A COOL DRY PLACE. FLAVOURED ELECTROLYTE DRINK. C INGREDIENTS: WATER, SUCROSE, GLUCOSE, FOOD ACID (330, 331), MONOPOTASSIUM PHOSPHATE, SODIUM CHLORIDE, FLAVOUR, COLOUR (133).

1. It shows the serving size is 600ml, and there is one serving in the package.
2. There are 9 ingredients in this drink with the second and third being sugar.
3. Scroll down the per serving column to the word sugar. It shows 36g of total sugar.
4. In looking at the ingredients closely. Flavour is concerning because we don't even know what is included in that. The colour 133 is called Brilliant Blue and when you look it up in chemical maze you will find it:

- Derived from petroleum
- Has quite a list of potential effects and symptoms – allergic reactions, asthma, may cause hyperactivity, suspected carcinogen, suspected mutagen, suspected neurotoxicity, skin ailments such as eczema and dermatitis. (source: Chemical Maze app)

I need to draw your attention to this colour blue 133 is not just used in this drink, it is used in most processed packaged foods that are blue. Cakes, lollies, icing and more.

Example 2: - BBQ Shapes

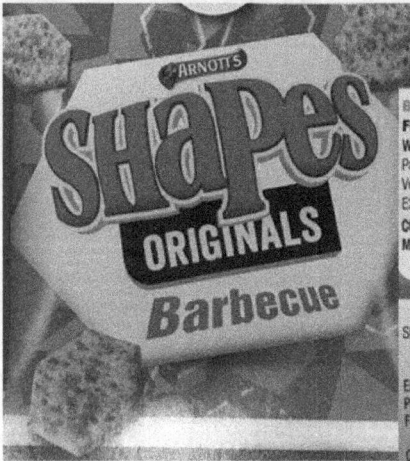

BBQ
FLAVOURED BISCUITS
Wheat Flour, Vegetable Oil, Starch (**Wheat**), Salt, Tomato Powder, Yeast, Garlic, Parsley, Sugar, Worcestershire Sauce, Onion Powder, Baking Powder, Natural Flavour, Vegetable Protein Extract (from Maize), Spices, Antioxidants (E300, E307b From Soy, E304), Flavour Enhancer (E635), Emulsifier (**Soy** Lecithin), Malt Extract (From Barley).
CONTAINS GLUTEN CONTAINING CEREALS AND SOY.
MAY CONTAIN TRACES OF EGG, MILK, PEANUT, SESAME AND TREE NUT.

NUTRITION INFORMATION
SERVINGS PER PACKAGE: 5   SERVING SIZE: 25 g

	QUANTITY PER SERVING	%DAILY INTAKE * (PER SERVING)	QUANTITY PER 100 g
ENERGY	515 kJ	5.9%	2,060 kJ
PROTEIN	1.9 g	3.8%	7.5 g
FAT, TOTAL	5.6 g	8.0%	22.4 g
-SATURATED	1.3 g	5.4%	5.2 g
CARBOHYDRATE	15.8 g	5.1%	63.4 g
-SUGARS	0.2 g	0.2%	0.9 g
DIETARY FIBRE	0.9 g	3.0%	3.4 g
SODIUM	171 mg	7.4%	685 mg

* BASED ON AN AVERAGE ADULT DIET OF 8700 KJ. ALL VALUES CONSIDERED AVERAGES UNLE

1. One lunchbox packet is 25g serving size
2. There are 20 ingredients, with salt being the 4th ingredient
3. In looking up the ingredients, you see there is Natural Flavour. We do not know what's in this particular flavour. Then I am going to jump straight to flavour enhancer 635. If this was to be listed with its name rather than the number it would be Disodium 5 – ribonucleotides. How many people do you

think have that in their pantry? When you look this up in the chemical maze app, you will find:

- It is banned in some countries
- The potential effects and symptoms are allergic reactions, behavioural problems, head ache, heart palpitations, should be avoided by asthmatics, hyperactivity, headaches and migraines, skin ailments like eczema and dermatitis.

Additives and Preservatives to Avoid

Look out for the additive and preservative numbers below. The ones listed in the table have been identified as the worst of each category by Francine Bell from Additive Free Kids. If you see any ingredients listed, it is recommended you avoid buying these foods. These have been identified as having a range of different effects such as behavioural issues, learning difficulties, hyperactivity, asthma, eczema, sleep disturbances and more.

Francine has developed a FREE guide for you that includes loads more information about these categories of additives. To get your copy, visit **Additive Free Kids** and download the FREE Additives To Avoid Guide.

Name	Numbers
Colours	102, 104, 110, 122, 123, 124, 127, 129, 132, 133, 142, 143, 150b, 150c, 150d, 151, 155, 160b, 171, 173
Preservatives	210, 211, 212, 213. 222, 223, 224, 225, 228, 249, 250, 251, 252, 280, 281, 283
Antioxidants	310, 311, 312, 319, 320, 321
Stabilisers/Thickeners	407 Carrageenan
Emulsifiers	431, 433, 435, 436
Flavour Enhancers	620, 621, 622, 623, 624, 625, 627, 631, 635
Acidity Regulators	acetates, acids, lactates, citrates, phosphates, malates, adipates, fumarates, pyrophosphates, sulphates, oxides.
Sweeteners	950, 951. 952, 954, 955, 961, 962

Recapping the five simple steps to reading the packet label

1. Ignore all the messages on the front of the item. Turn the packet around
2. Find the ingredient's list and Count the number of ingredients. if there is more than 6, consider putting the product back on the shelf and finding a more appropriate choice.
3. If sugar, salt or fat is listed in first 3 ingredients, put the product back on the shelf and find a more appropriate choice.
4. Calculate the number of teaspoons of sugar per serve
5. Look up each of the additives in The Chemical Maze app or a similar resource

Please do your family a favour and start making this a habit. Use this book as a starting point but please do your own research. Get your kids involved and teach them this. Food label literacy is a life skill everyone now needs to have. Processed food is firmly entrenched in our food culture now, so we have to be wise to what we buy.

How to Start Reading Packet Labels as a Habit.

The key is not to make this hard work. Change your headspace that this is about saving you time at the doctors later on in life or about giving your family more vitality. Or perhaps saving some of the behavioural arguments that go on at home or even getting more sleep. Yep, reducing the amount of processed food you eat could do any, some or more of these things for your family.

To keep this simple, it is suggested you do not try to read and change all your products at once. You may like to follow the process below:

1. Jot down a list of the top three processed foods you buy each week.
2. Next time you shop, turn the packets (jars, boxes, sachets etc) around and read the ingredients.
3. Make your judgement call about whether you want to keep buying this, finding a better one from the shelf or finding a recipe to make it at home.
4. Whenever you shop, shop consciously and enjoy the choices you make.
5. The next time you shop for these three processed foods, use the conscious choice you made when you read the labels the last time.
6. When these conscious choices are a way of life in your household, start the process again. What are the next three processed foods you buy regularly?

What we want to do is make this as easy as possible for you. If you don't want to do this at the supermarket, we live in an incredible world of the internet. You can sit down at your computer and can most often find out the ingredients without leaving home. Coles Online or Woolworths Online are wonderful resources. You type in the product in their search function and most times, you will find the ingredients list and nutritional information. Some of the manufacturers also list the ingredients on their websites too.

As a final caveat, I should say from time to time, manufacturers do change their product formulations, so it is important a couple of times a year to turn the packets around on the products you have already looked at. Check the ingredients are the same.

A Simple Way to Talk to Your Children

At various points in this book, I have shared different ways to talk to your kids about food and how it makes their bodies feel. If you've been doing this, then they will be starting to understand why we need to ask the question of "What's In My Food?"

I'd like to suggest you do a few things at this point:
1. Teach them how to read the packet label using the five steps you've just learnt.
2. Get them involved in reading the labels. You can do this from home too.

You don't need to continually say "no" when the kids ask you for something you'd prefer them not to have. Simply ask them; "What's in that food?" Then let them find out and tell you whether or not it's going to help their "One Body For Life."

You may be thinking: "Bel has gone stark raving mad. Do you know how long shopping is going to take if I have to turn over the packets plus get my kids involved too?"

But here's the thing, you don't even have to leave home to work out "What's In My Food?" You can look it up online. Screens are usually a weakness for most children, so use this to your advantage. Get them involved in looking up the products ingredients online.

Empower Your Kids with Screens

Technology can be used for good. Most kids love the opportunity to be on a screen so we can use this to our advantage when it comes to teaching kids how to read packet labels. You know your children better than anyone else. You determine which method of using screens will work for them.

Older children who are more independent on screens.

(Maybe 10 and above, who know how to type into a search function).

1. Show them how to use Coles or Woolworths Online, or Google the manufacturer to look up the ingredients.
2. Give them some products to review and show them how to use the Chemical Maze or similar book / app to look up the additives and preservatives.
3. Ask them to follow the five steps and to write down Yes foods and No foods.
4. Let them know together you will look at the Yes foods with them and together agree if you'll still buy them. For the No foods, together you'll work out if you are going to look for alternatives, make them at home or go without.

Younger children, who need more help on screens

(You will need to do the searching and have more playful conversations about what you see).

1. Sit them down right alongside you and tell them, "We're going to have some fun finding out what's in our food."
2. Use Coles or Woolworths Online to look up the products and use the five steps.

3. Ask your kids to count on their fingers as you say the ingredients.

4. When you finished saying them, ask them how many fingers did we count then? Was it more than six?

5. If it was more than six, say something like, "Mmm, there's a lot of ingredients in that. Maybe it's not the best one for our one body for life." Put it aside in the No pile.

6. When using the Chemical Maze app to look up additives and preservatives, use the smiley face pictures to get your child involved. If it's a sad face, you can say, "Oh, that's a sad face. Do you think we should be putting this in our body if it's a sad face?" Kids are smarter than we give them credit for. They are likely to shake their head and say "no". Put it in the No pile. If it has a happy face, then you can share with them it's a happy face and if it's passed the other steps, you can put it in the Yes pile.

Stop Saying No

Kids love a power struggle with their parents. Saying No is almost like an invitation for them to nag you to have it or to find someone that will give them some anyway. Instead of saying no, say "I don't know what's in it. Turn the packet around and have a look at the ingredients. Let's have a look at what's in it, then we can decide."

By doing this, you're not saying no. You're educating them that before you buy something, you turn the packet around and read the ingredients. Ask them to decide if they want to eat that for their One Body For Life. You are giving them life skills they will need – and use – for the rest of their life.

Your kids will turn the packet around, and they will look at the ingredients. The goal from all of this is to get your kids to be self-selecting not to have some of these foods. It's way better than you having to argue about why you don't want them to have it and it's teaching them a skill they will have for life.

This can go a couple of different ways. They look at the ingredients and say forget it, nope I don't want to eat that. Trust me this does happen and it's a wonderful feeling.

Or they may say, I know it's got heaps of ingredients and sugar in it, but I just want to have it anyway. Just so you know, this still happens with our kids occasionally despite the fact we have been doing this for almost nine years. When this happens, and it will, remember these foods are specifically formulated and marketed to get people to want them even when they know they aren't great for them. Use it as another chance for education, not argument.

If they are saying they really want to have a product even after reading the label and they know it's not good for them, remain calm and have a rational conversation with them. Have a chat about the ingredients and break the ingredients down with them. Talk about the number of ingredients. How heavily processed is it? Talk about the amount of sugar. How does that compare to the amount that's recommended for the day? Talk about the additives and preservatives. Talk about what else are they likely to eat in the day when they have this. Get them to think about the picture of all their food for the day. Talk about the impact buying this food may have not just on their body, but on the environment and wild life too.

At this point, please remember you are the parent. You have the final say. Do not give your power away. I like to recommend you set your own boundaries. For instance, when it comes to additives and preservatives, which ones are you going to make a hard no, and which ones are you okay with as having sometimes. And when I say sometimes, I am talking occasionally, every now again, irregularly etc.

To give you an example, I personally steer clear of any additive or preservative linked to behavioural problems, learning, and sleep disturbance because I don't wish to be dealing with these. Being a parent is hard enough. Any food which contains an additive or preservative which is listed as a suspected carcinogen, suspected mutagen, or suspected neurotoxicity is a hard NO for me. The fact it's suspected means research has shown inconclusively there is a chance. Just like with tobacco all those years ago, it can take a lot of years to prove or disprove that chance. I prefer not to let my kids be a guinea pig for that chance. I just don't want to risk it.

Set your own boundaries. Let them know your boundaries. And say something like, no amount of pleading will change my mind on this one. It is my job as your parent to keep you safe. I am not prepared to let you have this until this is proven safe.

It's also important to teach your kids to set their own boundaries. Once you have shared what's in food, ask them to think about what they definitely do not want to be putting into their bodies.

The most powerful "no" to a processed food, is the "no" your kids make. Educate and empower them to make better choices for their body, and you'll be giving them the skills for life.

Real Life Examples of This in Practice

We rarely buy packet lunchbox food, but it doesn't stop our kids from asking for it sometimes. Here's a couple of examples of how I get my kids involved in making the choice about whether to put food in our shopping trolley.

Cheese sticks

One day when I was shopping with our then eight-year-old son, he begged me to have Bega Cheese Sticks. He told me he had already looked at the ingredients and they had the exact same thing in them as the block of Bega Cheese we buy. I said, "Okay mate, let Mum have a look." And he was right. The exact same ingredients. Inwardly, I didn't want to buy them as they are so uneconomical compared to buying a block and cutting it into sticks myself, but I am conscious it's important for our kids to feel like they fit in. I agreed to buy them because ingredient-wise they were fine.

He was so excited as he put them in the trolley. However, I also used it as an opportunity to educate too. As we were walking around, we had a chat about those cheese sticks. It went something like this:

Me: "*Thanks for reading the ingredients. Mum didn't realise they were the same as what was in the block. When you eat one this week, what will you do with the wrapper?*"

Mr 8: "*Put it in the rubbish bin.*"

Me: "*Where do you think it will go after the rubbish bin?*"

Mr 8: "*It will get collected by the garbage truck and it'll end up in landfill.*"

Me: "*How long do you think it will last in landfill or do you think there's a chance it could blow away and make its way into our waterways?*"

Mr 8: "*It's plastic, so it's going be around for a lot of years and it could blow away I guess.*"

Me: "*Mmm, even though the ingredients in those sticks are okay for your body, perhaps it's not really a good choice for the environment. What do you think?*"

Mr 8: "*Not really.*"

Me: "*I agree. How about we have them this time, and we wait for a long time before we choose to have them again?*"

Mr 8: "*Okay, Mum.*"

Empowering our kids with knowledge and getting them involved in the decision making is so powerful. In this example, he got his cheese sticks but was gently reminded what might be an okay choice for his body was not necessarily a great choice for the environment. He learnt Mum will sometimes say yes, and he also learnt this yes does not mean every week.

Blocks of Chicken 2-Minute Noodles

Oh, this story makes me laugh at the logic of a tween. Our then eleven-year-old daughter and I were out shopping for groceries. She was in Year 7 at the time and going through a period of not eating much of her lunch at school but demolishing it at home. Evidently at school, Year 7 girls don't really eat much and what they do eat, is on the run and it's not real food.

On the drive, she'd been telling me about how all the girls were eating those blocks of noodles. I listened asking the normal questions. Do you think that's good for their body, how do they concentrate in class? etc). When I was in one of the aisles, she came up to me with a bag with multiple packs of the noodles in them. She was excited and said, "Mum, this is what the girls are eating. Can we buy some?

Here's how I handled this:

Me: "Sweetie, you know what, why don't you turn the packet around and look at the ingredients, then we can talk about it."

Miss 11: She turned the packet around and read the ingredients aloud. Her response was, "Oh Mum, it's rubbish. I know it is, but can we still buy them."

Me: Rather than say no outright, I wanted her to get to this point herself so I said, "You know what, if you want them that badly, you can use your pocket money to buy them."

Miss 11: "I am not going to waste my money on this rubbish."

Me: "Well, why would you think I would waste our family's food budget on that rubbish?"

Miss 11: Silence, then "Okay" as she puts them back on the shelf.

In this case, I didn't say an outright no, but she knew I was not going to buy them.

---

*Every request is an opportunity to empower
and educate our kids.*

Chapter 12
What to Pack in Your Child's Lunchbox

B y now you could be forgiven for thinking "Well, what the bleep do I pack in my kids lunchbox now?"

Lunchboxes are Super Important.

30-40% of what your children will eat Monday to Friday comes from what you pack in their lunchbox. When you send your kids to school with a lunchbox, you are effectively outsourcing every aspect of them – their growth, development, concentration, behaviour, ability to socialise and learn – to their teachers and their school. The fuel you pack in their lunchbox is what will help them do all this.

But here's the thing. Lunchboxes do not need to be difficult. In fact, they can be simple. The challenge is, simple does not always equal easy if your children are used to packet laden lunchboxes. Putting this aside, let's look at how simple they can be.

Outlined below I have included a fundamental rule of our lunchbox eCourse which helps busy parents pack healthy lunchboxes in about five minutes a day. If you follow this rule, you can feel confident in knowing you have packed your child a lunchbox which will support them to be the best version of themselves they can be at school.

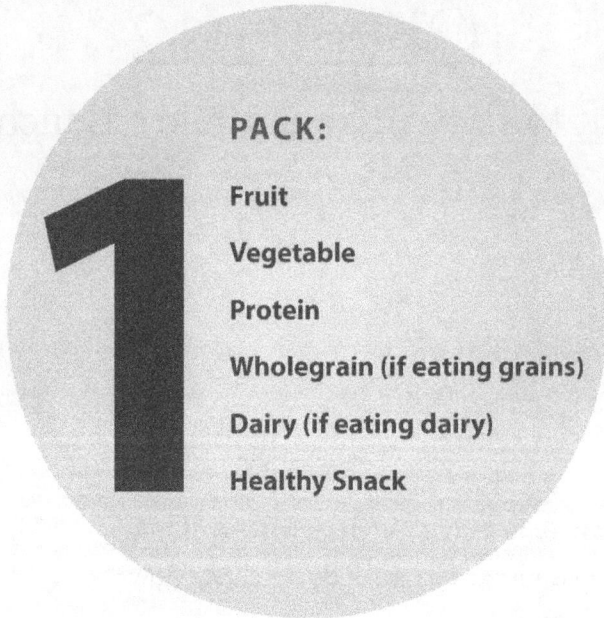

PACK:

Fruit

Vegetable

Protein

Wholegrain (if eating grains)

Dairy (if eating dairy)

Healthy Snack

See, simple. But achieving this is not always easy. This is because processed food, particularly in school lunchboxes has become normalised and through marketing, we have been led to believe this is what we pack into lunchboxes.

Most processed lunchbox foods are empty in nutrients and do very little to keep children's tummies full. That's one reason parents pack more than one packet, because they know when they eat them at home, they are still hungry afterwards.

In this chapter, we will cover in more depth what to pack in your child's lunchbox. If your child is used to having packet foods in the lunchbox, then you will need to have conversations about why this needs to change. Keep in mind, the simplest thing you can start to do start right now is:

1. Ask your kids what fruit and vegetables they want in this week's lunchbox and pack them.
2. Reduce the number of packets you currently include. If you normally pack two, pack more fruit and vegetables and pack only one packet food. If you normally pack three packets, pack two and more fruit and vegetables.

With only around 6% of Australian children eating the recommended amounts of fruits and vegetables, it is important to start getting a little more not just in their lunchbox but in their other meals too. If you leave all the five serves of vegetables for the dinner plate, that's a lot of vegetables required to be eaten at dinner.

Here's a tip, every time you serve a meal (including breakfast) or a snack, think, "How can I add a small amount of vegetables to this?" Grated carrot and grated zucchini are simple options to add and can even be added to porridge or overnight oats.

Now, back to lunchboxes. Outlined here is a way to chat to your children about their lunchboxes and more detailed information for you to pack.

A Simple Way to Talk to Your Children

NAQ (previously Nutrition Australia Queensland) developed this simple concept to help to remember kids understand how foods keep them healthy. You can use this to help pack lunchboxes by breaking the foods into Go, Glow and Grow Foods.

GO Foods	
Food Type	A mix of long lasting carbohydrates and good quality fats.
Purpose	This is our body's and brain's fuel. These foods help us play and concentrate.
Examples	Carbohydrate are wholegrain breads and pastas, rice, quinoa, oats, legumes. Good Fat are butter, cheese, avocado, oily fish like tuna and salmon.

GROW Foods	
Food Type	Quality proteins
Purpose	Helps build bones, muscles, teeth and keeps tummies fuller for longer which helps brains stay focussed.
Examples	Proteins are chicken, beef, turkey, egg, tuna, salmon, fish, tofu, tempeh, legumes (chickpeas, kidney beans etc), nuts (If your school allows them). *Note, quality protein does not include processed meats like ham.*

GLOW Foods	
Food Type	Rich in fibre, vitamins and minerals.
Purpose	Helps our skin, hair, eyes and importantly, assists the immune system to stay strong.
Examples	Fruits and vegetables are glow foods. Different colours of fruits and vegetables can help different parts of the body. Eating a rainbow of fruits and vegetables everyday helps.

A Deeper Chat for Adults

When we travelled, we saw many lunchboxes and spoke to many teachers and parents. One of the biggest things we noticed about school lunchbox food was that it was heavy on the carbohydrates.

These carbohydrates are mostly coming from lunchbox packet foods and white bread, so they are largely empty carbohydrates. What this means is the lunchboxes create a spike in energy, but this energy is short lived. To sustain our children for a whole day at school, a balanced lunchbox is required.

A balanced lunchbox includes a mix of carbohydrates, proteins and good fats. Let's take a look at each one of these in more detail.

Carbohydrates

Carbohydrates are one of our body's main sources of energy so undeniably they are important. They are made up of fibre, starch and sugar. However, not all carbohydrates are equal.

One of the most important things to remember about carbohydrates is they all ultimately breakdown to sugar. What sets the different carbohydrates apart is their fibre component. A carbohydrate that contains a higher amount of fibre compared to starch and sugar are the ones we need to be putting in their lunchbox. This is because the fibre makes our body digest the food more slowly, which means the sugar doesn't get released in a big spike. The amount of fibre is particularly important because the more fibre, the fuller it will help our kids stay plus it also helps with bowel movements. The types of carbohydrates needed in a lunchbox tend to be called complex carbohydrates, and they are found in:

- Fruits
- Vegetables
- Nuts (if you're school allows nuts)
- Seeds (like pepitas and sunflower)
- Beans - navy beans, kidney beans, black beans, cannellini beans, chickpeas
- Wholegrains (brown rice, buckwheat, barley, millet, oatmeal, popcorn, whole-wheat bread, pasta, quinoa)

When it comes to your grains, remember the whiter the product is, the more processed it is. Wholegrains are darker in colour because they retain the three parts of their original seed (the bran, germ and endosperm) and contain better sources of fibre and other important nutrients. When choosing bread, you need to make sure you see wholegrains in the top three ingredients, preferably the first ingredient.

Proteins

Bodies require protein for growth and development. If you think about this logically, when does most growth happen? In our childhood years. Our children's bodies require protein because they are growing so rapidly.

Our body requires protein to make hair, skin, nails, feel good hormones, and reproductive hormones. It's needed to build new cells. If that's not important enough, our body can't actually store protein, so for our body to build and repair we need to be eating protein.

Aside from the importance to the growth and development of our children's body, protein also helps keep tummies full.

Some signs your child may not be getting enough protein include:
* Getting sick frequently,
* Poor muscle strength,
* And even having a poor appetite.

Include a small amount of protein for both recess and main lunch if you can. Protein can be from plant sources or animal sources and can be included in the following ways.
* Chicken. Do not underestimate the power of how you can use a roast chicken.
* Good quality mincemeat – make it into hamburgers, meatball subs, Spag Bolognese, lasagna and more.
* Roast beef, lamb.

- Chickpeas – in a salad, make hummus, falafel balls, in a salad, serve as a finger food.
- Cheese – cube it, grate it, slice it, include it on a sandwich.
- Plain yoghurt – preferably Greek Yoghurt.
- Eggs. What can't you do with eggs? Boil them, mash them for a sandwich filling, make an omelette style wrap and more.
- Tuna – add to sandwiches, mix with cream cheese to make a dip.
- Seeds – pepitas, sunflower, sesame. Make them into a trail mix, turn them into a muesli bar, add them to breads.
- Homemade baked beans – wraps, corn chips.
- Lentils and other beans.
- Tofu, tempeh.

Just a couple of notes about meats. Deli meats such as ham, and salami are not the best source of protein, plus they are usually laced with sugar and preservatives. The common preservative is nitrate. Remember to read the packet label or ask the deli for the ingredients list. Also, wherever possible, try to source meat and poultry where the animal has been raised ethically and fed well. It is important to realise, whatever the animal has been fed, and however the animal has been treated, becomes part of what we eat. With that said, I am a firm believer that you do the best with the budget you have and if going from a deli meat to a whole chicken you cook yourself is the best your budget and time can stretch to, then that's a mighty fine start.

Fats
The brain is our fattiest organ, and it's estimated it's made up of about 60% fat. The brain needs fat to help the neurons talk to other neurons. This means fat is important to memory and our cognitive function. But like we've spoken about already, the fat needs to be good fats. Saturated fats and trans fats, are considered inferior for the brain. They can slow down the processing of information and overall brain

function. The quality of the fats can also have an impact on mood and the balance of our emotions. [66]

The types of fats important for our brain are called Omega-3 fats. They are found in foods like:

- Avocado
- Olive oil
- Nuts - walnuts are particularly good for brains. Notice how they even look like a brain.
- Seeds
- Fatty fish
- Flaxseeds
- Chia seeds
- Algae

Small amounts of saturated fats from coconut oil, grass fed meats and butter and ghee have also been suggested as valuable for brain function.[67]

The fats found in processed foods are not great for brain health. They can lead to poor memory function, inflammation in the brain and even longer term brain issues such as Dementia and Alzheimer's disease. Look out for the words: saturated, trans fats, hydrogenated, partially hydrogenated oils and even vegetable oils because these go through a very long refining process involving "extraction, chemical solvents, sodium hydroxide (lye), high pressure and heat, filtration, bleaching, chemical treatment and deodorising." [68]

If you look at the ingredients of processed lunchbox foods, you will find vegetable oils is used extensively. They are a cheap ingredient and as long as the oil doesn't come from an animal, it can be called vegetable oil. It could be made from one or a combination of corn, canola, soy, peanut, olive, sesame, safflower, coconut, sunflower, cottonseed or palm oil. This generic term "vegetable oil" doesn't tell us anything about what's actually in it, where it has come from nor how it was produced..

Our brain needs both Omega-3 and Omega-6 fatty acids, but there needs to be a balance of between 2:1 to 4:1 of Omega-3's to Omega-6's. Unfortunately, Omega-6 acids are abundant in vegetable oils. The increase in the amount of processed foods being consumed today that use vegetable oils means there has been a significant increase in the consumption of Omega-6.

Researchers have hypothesized this increase of Omega-6 corresponds to the increase in the rate of overweight and obesity in adults.[69] If they have hypothesized this for adults, what does it mean to children who are eating these packet foods containing vegetable oil every day in their lunchbox?

What Makes a Great Sandwich?

As we travelled Australia, it was clear a sandwich is still the most common main lunch for most children. But not all sandwiches are equal. What makes a great sandwich that will keep your child full and support their learning comes from the quality of the three components of a sandwich. Each are important.

1. Bread
2. Spread
3. Filling

A white bread sandwich with margarine and vegemite or honey, jam or Nutella is not a great sandwich. It creates a spike in energy followed by a crash. There is little nutrition in any of those ingredients.

On the other hand, a good quality whole grain bread, with real butter, avocado, tahini, nut butters (if allowed) or homemade mayonnaise as the spread, with a filling of protein (e.g. chicken, egg, cheese, chickpeas) is far superior.

If you're thinking "There is no way I could get my child to eat a sandwich like that," then just remember you do not have to change everything at once. Ask yourself, what can I do to make the sandwich I pack today a little more nutritious? Here's some simple swaps:

Food	Simple Swap
White bread	Wholegrain. You could even take this slower by having one piece of white bread, the other wholegrain.
Margarine	Real butter. I realise many guidelines from authorities still recommend margarine but take a look at the ingredients. They are highly processed.
Vegemite	Add some lettuce or cheese
Honey	Change to raw honey or honey bought from a bee farmer. Most supermarket honey is highly processed and lost nutritional value. Add some banana or cream cheese or even chicken. This will make the sandwich more filling and slow down the use of the sugar in the honey.
Jam	Trade store bought jam to homemade chia jam Check out my recipe for chia jam on our website. Trade jam for a banana sandwich or add some sunflower butter or tahini plus the jam. What we're trying to do is slow down all that sugar in jam.

Make small changes. You don't have to do these swaps all at once. Maybe make your focus on improving the bread first. Or the filling. You know your family better than anyone else. What is likely to give you the quickest win in adding more nutrition?

Get your kids involved in building more nutritious sandwiches by grabbing your FREE Bonus How To Build A Great Sandwich Template.

Grab your FREE Bonuses for The Lunchbox Effect:
http://thelunchboxeffect.com/bonuses

Lunchbox Ideas

In most of the schools we visited around Australia, children get about ten minutes to eat their lunch. This means the food we pack not only needs to be nutritious but easy to eat too.

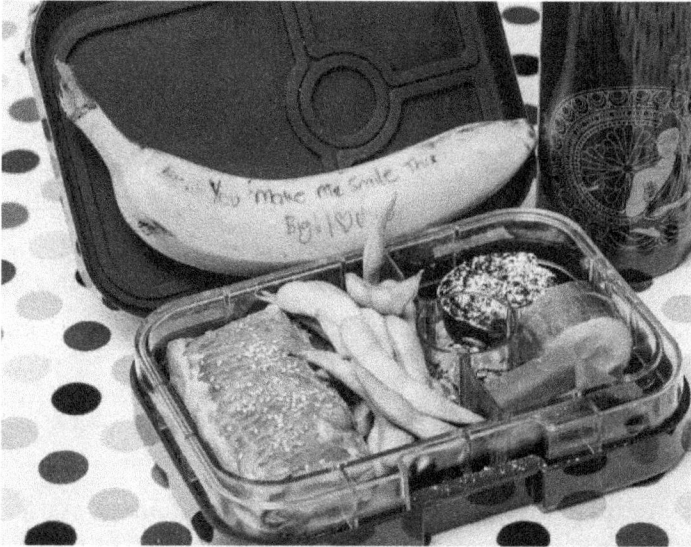

A very simple but balanced lunchbox could contain:
- A chicken or egg, lettuce and cheese sandwich using wholegrain bread with avocado, good quality butter or homemade mayonnaise as the spread.
- A piece of fruit.
- Some veggie sticks and a dip. (e.g. hummus)
- A homemade snack or a packet that you have consciously chosen from the supermarket

In our work, parents often tell us they don't have time to pack real food or the packet foods are packed as a snack or a "treat" for their kids. Below is a list of simple real foods snacks that are quick to pack.

• Cherry tomatoes • Fruit salad • Plain crackers with cheese or dips • Bliss balls • Plain Greek yoghurt, top with muesli or fruit • Popcorn popped at home	• Baby cucumbers • Veggie sticks (carrot, cucumber, tomato, celery) and a dip • Berries, grapes • Edamame (hummus) • Cheese cubes/sticks cut from a block of cheese • Homemade biscuit / slice

Some of these may require a little bit of preparation on the weekend but this time will set you up for a week. Now I am going to be bold here, if you think you don't have time, then I encourage you to think about how you spend time. If there is time to mindlessly scroll through Facebook or Instagram looking at what others are up to, then trading this time with a little preparation so you can pack more nourishing food in your child's lunchbox is a worthwhile trade.

Look, the honest truth of the matter is this. Anything you make at home, from wholefood ingredients (not a packet mix) will be superior in terms of nutrition to what comes from a packet from the supermarket. Even if you make good old fashioned biscuits or cakes using white flour, butter and sugar, they would still be better because there are no additives.

I cannot stress this enough. As a parent or guardian, you have the power to immediately control what goes into your child's lunchbox. You don't have to wait for the government to issue guidelines, you don't need me to tell you. This is in your control. I know this may sound challenging and may require a headspace shift, but lunchboxes do not need to be complicated. They have been made complicated by food manufacturers, advertising and supermarket displays telling us these foods are convenient, perfect for lunchboxes and constantly reminding us that we are too busy. Hopefully you can see from this, it's not complicated. If we put our children's health and education as a priority, then we can always find time to do a bit of preparation to ensure they have healthy nourishing lunchboxes.

Get your kids involved in helping to pack their own lunchbox by using my simple visual template of the 5 Steps to Pack a Healthy Lunchbox.

Grab your FREE Bonuses for The Lunchbox Effect:
http://thelunchboxeffect.com/bonuses

Simple Packet Swaps

Remember this book isn't about saying no to packet food, it's about eating more fruits and vegetables, and minimising processed packet foods. If you want to include processed packet foods in the lunchbox, then ask What's In My Food – choose the packet consciously.

Here are some simple swaps you may wish to consider. Please remember to still read the ingredients list even of these swaps. A better swap for all of these in the table is just to pack more fresh fruit and vegetables.

Packet	Swap To	From the shops	Make at home
Flavoured Chips	→	Plain chips and plain rice crackers.	Gluten Free Cracker Recipe
Flavoured Crackers	→	Plain air popped popcorn or plain rice crackers.	Homemade Popcorn (Kids will love it!)
Juice Boxes	→	Water plus Whole / cut piece of fruit	
Muesli Bars	→	Plain Pikelets (not the flavoured shake and bake)	Homemade Pikelets (Great for brekky too!)
Chocolates or lollies	→	Bliss Balls	Chocolate Protein Bomb Bliss Balls
Yoghurt tubs / pouches	→	Natural yoghurt and flavour with frozen fruit pureed	

Recipes
- Gluten Free Cracker Recipe: **http://rootcau.se/gfcrackers**
- Homemade Popcorn: **http://rootcau.se/popcorn**
- Homemade Pikelets: **http://rootcau.se/pikelets**
- Chocolate Protein Bombs: **http://rootcau.se/chocbombs**

There's always time for what we make our priority. If we make our children's health a priority, we will find the time.

For more free lunchbox ideas, follow us on social media:
Facebook: **https://www.facebook.com/theRootCauseAU**
Instagram: **@theRootCauseAU**

Real Food is Too Expensive

This is a common complaint by many parents. Food manufacturers have done a great job telling us processed food is convenient and cheaper than real food. When you really start to look at it, you will find in many cases real food is as affordable as processed foods, and sometimes even cheaper. You can't get much simpler than adding fruit and some cut up vegetables to a lunchbox. Even when you need to do some preparation, this can often be done ahead of time.

Let's look at some cost comparison examples: (prices taken from Woolworths Online at Dec 2019)

Packaged "Lunchbox" Foods		Real Food Examples	
6 x Woolworths Fruit Drink 250ml	$2.65	1kilo Odd Bunch Green Apples (approx. 6 small apples)	$3.00
6pk Uncle Toby's Muesli Bars (equates to 71cents)	$4.30	1kilo Cavendish Bananas	$3.90
70g Pauls Strawberry Yoghurt Pouch	$1.40	70g Homemade Strawberry Yoghurt	$1.87*
		• Tamar Valley Natural Green Yoghurt 1kg	$6.20
		• 250g Strawberry Punnet	$4.00
		• 10px Sinchies Reusable Pouches	$16.00
		Total	$26.20
		*The ingredients listed will make 14 serves of Homemade Strawberry Yoghurt, plus you can re-use the pouches. Equates to $1.87 each serve.	

NSW Health have created a great video to help illustrate how eating healthy doesn't have to be more expensive. It's called "Swap It – The Cost of Healthy Living" and you can watch it here: **http://rootcau.se/swapitvideo**

If you want more help with how to pack healthy, packet-free lunchboxes for your child, I created an online course – The 5 Minute Healthy Lunchbox System – which teaches exactly that. It helps you put systems in place to make real food lunches easy, affordable and fast for your child's lunchbox. Learn more here: **https://therootcause.com.au/lunchbox**

Chapter 13
Start Asking "What's In My Food?"

The Root Cause at the end of 2018 requested their community ask their children what are three the most common lunchbox packets foods they see at school. For ease, they have been grouped into product categories from order of most common to least. There are obviously other lunchbox products outside these categories, but these were the ones which children said they saw at school.

I was legitimately shocked by the number of processed packet lunchbox foods there were. Please note, this is by no means an exhaustive list of foods dressed up for school lunchboxes. When the idea of this book was conceived, it is fair to say the sheer volume of products available was underestimated. The contributors to this book have learnt to live without these foods for their families. Suffice to say, we have been totally shocked by the sheer number of products available.

You will note we have also included breads and wraps as a category. This is because sandwiches are a staple main lunch for most children. When we asked, "What's In Our Food?" for breads and wraps, we were amazed by the number of ingredients. Given the importance a sandwich plays in the lunchbox, we thought you should gain an understanding of what's in breads and wraps too.

In compiling this information, we did our absolute best to get this information right for you. We must report it was significantly more difficult than we realised. Some of the lists of ingredients are so long they needed to be counted three, sometimes more times, to work out how many there were. It should also be remembered all we counted and recorded here for the purpose of this book, is the ingredients listed. We know some ingredients are made up of other ingredients, such as flavours, but we have absolutely no idea how many or what they are, so we couldn't possibly count them.

It was also a lot more difficult than we expected to work out the number of additives because manufacturers can choose when to use the number assigned by FSANZ or to use words, and sometimes those words aren't always clear they are an additive.

In terms of sugar and the number of teaspoons of sugar, it is important to remember that this is all sugar, not just the free sugar referred to by WHO as being what we need to look out for. Currently, Australian labelling laws do not require free sugar to be listed out separately. Be aware though if sugar (or one of the sixty plus names used for it) is listed as an ingredient, then it is free sugar (been added by the manufacturer). If it is in the top three ingredients, then it's a major part of the product.

This chapter outlines the details by product category. This information allows you to get a helicopter view of what's in the average product within a product category. You can use this information to draw your own conclusions about whether you want to continue including this product category in the lunchbox. Or spend more time reviewing the individual products in the appendix and in the Online

Product Companion. You may also to choose to find a recipe to make at home or decide you simply don't need this sort of food.

In the following chapter, you will find the information detailed for the individual products we reviewed.

The Data Explained

The following table shows the product category reviewed and the average amounts of ingredients, teaspoons of sugar, where sugar (or sweetener) is in the top three ingredients. It also includes the additives and the sum of the number of products per category that contain additives with the potential effects listed in the table.

How to Read the Table

Let's take muesli bars because they are the most common packet in lunchboxes according to the survey of children by parents in the community. Please remember, this data is based on serving size – not 100g. This is intentional so you can see what your child would be eating in one packet.

Muesli bars – we reviewed eighty-seven varieties. On average they had:
- 24.3 ingredients
- Two teaspoons of sugar
- Sugar is in the top three ingredients
- 8.1 additives
- The number of products that included additives with potential effects of: Learning difficulties were possible from two products, behavioural problems from two products, hyperactivity from eleven, depression from five, headaches from sixty, asthma from thirty-four, sleep disturbance from seven, and twenty-five could contribute to eczema.

What you can take from this is that on average muesli bars are heavily processed and contain a significant proportion of the WHO recommended amount of sugar for the **entire day**, not just one snack. Sugar appears in the top 3 three ingredients on average so is a major ingredient in the average muesli bar. If you have a child who is hyperactive, has headaches, asthma, sleep disturbance or eczema, you may wish to reconsider whether the average muesli bar is a good option for their one body for life.

With this knowledge, you may choose to:
- Keep packing muesli bars in the lunchbox
- Not pack muesli bars in the lunchbox at all
- Pack them only sometimes
- Keep them for home
- Make them a sometimes food at home
- Find a recipe to make them at home (choosing whether it will be a sometimes or everyday food)
- Go without muesli bars
- Do more research of the individual muesli products and choose one you are happy with (choosing whether it will be a sometimes or everyday food)

Summary by Product Category

Product category	No. Products Reviewed	Avg No. of Ingredients	Avg No. of Additives	Avg Sugar (g)	Avg Sugar (tsp)	Sugar in Top 3?	Avg Sodium (mg)
Chips	91	12.4	3.4	0.7	0.15	No	128.9
Muesli & Other Bars	92	24.3	8.1	8.2	2	Yes	46.5
Savoury Crackers	56	16.9	5.2	0.9	0.2	No	166
Sweet Biscuits	34	18.2	5.8	9.1	2.3	Yes	67
Juice & Flavoured Milks	61	7.6	2.8	22	5.5	No	30
Yoghurt Tubs & Pouches	82	12	4.2	12	3	Yes	41.6
Chocolate & Lollies	24	15.7	5.5	10.1	2.5	Yes	11.2
Fruit & Jelly Cups	15	10.4	6.8	18.2	4.6	Yes	41.4
Bread & Wraps	65	17	3.5	2.5	0.6	No	291

Sum of Potential Effects

Product category	Learning Difficulties	Behaviour	Hyperactivity	Depression	Headache/Migraine	Asthma	Sleep Disturbance	Eczema/Skin Conditions
Chips	40	44	21	40	44	44	17	32
Muesli & Other Bars	2	2	11	5	60	34	7	25
Savoury Crackers	1	11	11	4	4	17	10	25
Sweet Biscuits	0	0	7	0	2	2	0	8
Juice & Flavoured Milks	0	0	8	0	4	9	0	8
Yoghurt Tubs & Pouches	1	1	4	1	1	12	1	4
Chocolate & Lollies	2	2	8	2	2	8	2	13
Fruit & Jelly Cups	0	0	2	0	0	2	0	2
Bread & Wraps	9	13	2	5	16	16	8	13

Chapter 14
Simple Actions You Can Take Right Now

Get Your Kids Involved

There are so many different ways to do this, so the list below is not exhaustive. You will find plenty of other ideas on the internet too.

1. Ask them

I know this sounds counter intuitive but when we make decisions for our kids, it's like we're imposing our thoughts and desires upon them. The simple question of "What fruits and vegetables would you like this week?" can make a massive difference to your child's acceptance of eating them. Even if they choose the same ones, focus on just slowly increasing the quantities of what they do like.

2. Have fun with it

Taking the stress out of getting your kids to try foods is really important – for you and for them. No one likes to change, so if you just put it on their plate and expect them to eat it, then you may be disappointed if they don't. If they come to the table feeling anxious because they are expecting you to "nag" them about eating their vegetables, they are less likely to eat it too. So have fun with it. Some ideas on how you can have fun are:

- **Pick Platters or Picnic Plates** – set up a big platter in the middle of the table with loads of different cut up vegetables and dips. Let your child take what they want and put it on their plate.

- **Muffin Trays** – fill the holes of the muffin tray with different colours of fruits or vegetables, or maybe have a theme colour day. For instance, a red day, so you fill the holes with different red fruits or vegetables.

- **The Crunch Game** – have a platter of different vegetables and get each person to go around and see who can make it crunch the loudest. Test out all of the vegetables on the platter. Keep score. Maybe the person who has the loudest crunch wins some experience (e.g. bowling, movie etc).

- **The Which Way Game** – In this game, you get the kids to choose a fruit or vegetable, then you prepare it in a number of different ways. Get the kids to try the different ways, asking them to use their senses (sight, smell, touch, sound, taste) and ask them to rate them. You could even use a simple taste test sheet where they circle happy or sad faces about how they like it. Of course, change this up depending on their age.

- **Food on a Stick** – This is usually always a winner. Make rainbow skewers, colour themed skewers, get the kids to make their own from a platter. Eat them raw, cook them on the BBQ, brush them with a marinade and cook.

3. Cook with them

Okay, so I know the reasons why not to cook with the kids. I don't have time. It gets too messy. It tests our patience. But there are many reasons why we *should* cook with our kids too. I've listed some below:

Cooking with our kids has so many important benefits such as:

- **Improved relationship with you** – I put this first because what happens when you're in the kitchen, guiding your child, but trusting them is something magical. You are close, you banter about anything and everything, you laugh, you celebrate – even the "epic fails".
- **Pride in themselves** – the smile that spreads across their face when they see what they made makes your heart melt. They are so proud of themselves.
- **More likely to try foods** – because they have been involved, it breaks down the fear around the food, and they are more likely to try foods they wouldn't have before.
- **Increased self-confidence** – every time they cook something, their self-confidence increases. They become more prepared and more excited to put themselves out there and try new things.
- **Increased self-esteem** – self achievement leads to improved belief in themselves.
- **Improved relationship to food** – choosing produce helps them understand about freshness, teaches them to look at where the produce is from, develops an appreciation for flavours, and a willingness to try foods.
- **The skill of following instructions** – this teaches them there is an order to do things, but it also teaches them to think out of the box too. For instance, if you don't have maple syrup, what else can you use instead.
- **Improved maths** – measurement, servings etc are all an opportunity to improve maths.

- **Shopping skills** – an understanding of what to look for in produce along with how much food costs.
- **Development of kitchen techniques** – understanding the difference between slicing and dicing, sautéing and simmering etc.
- **Understanding culture** – different meals may come from different cultures / countries. It's an opportunity to look at where these countries are and why these foods are popular there.
- **Improved appreciation of parents** – our kids learn what it takes to turn out a meal for breakfast, lunch and dinner. They realise it's not instantaneous, that it takes effort and love to make it happen.

So get cooking with the kids. This could be as simple as getting them to add flour or helping them cook a whole meal. One of the biggest gifts you can give your children is the love of real food and enjoying preparing meals with it. You should aim to teach your kids to get themselves breakfast, pack their own lunch and ultimately be able to cook at least one meal a week. When you do this, you will not just be giving them life skills but taking away some of your workload too.

4. Make food colourful and fun

It is true, most people taste food with their eyes first. It's one of the secrets to marketing of processed foods. It's why the packaging is so bright and colourful to attract the attention of the kids and us too. So we need to match this technique. We need to make our food colourful and fun. It's not that difficult given nature provides us with so many delicious fruits and vegetables from all the colours of the rainbow.

When you're preparing food, think about the colours on the plate. I always strive to have at least three different colours of fruits and vegetables in the meals and snacks I serve. Most days I make that, some days I don't but that's the goal. Colourful so it looks attractive when you serve it.

Fun can be as simple as the banter you have at the table. It could be pick plates where they get to choose. It could be build it meals – where you have a host of different fillings in the centre of the table and they get to build their own burger, wrap, pizza, rice paper roll, etc. Or you could even serve food up on a plate in the shape of a face. There are so many ways to have fun with food.

5. Family Meals and Rituals

In today's busy world, the whole family sitting down to a meal together has become more difficult. However, there are so many benefits. Studies have shown benefits are quite profound such as:

- Better academic performance
- Greater resilience
- Higher self-esteem
- Lower likelihood of depression
- Lower likelihood of developing an eating disorder

It is suggested that you carve out at least a couple of times a week where you can have a meal together. This does not have to be the evening meal. It could be breakfast, or it could be snacks. The goal is for _**several**_ family meals, where the whole family comes together, is seated around the table, conversing with each other, no TV/ phones/ technology, each and every week.

Creating family rituals around food is a great way of bringing some fun to eating together too. For instance, we do Sunday Family Day Pancakes. Sometimes I make them, sometimes Israel, and sometimes our thirteen-year-old daughter will make them. Soon we will teach our nine-year-old son to make them. But regardless of who makes them, we always have them on Sunday morning. Sometimes we even get organised and take the batter down to the beach and cook them on the BBQ, so we eat our pancakes looking out at the water.

We also have Fun Family Friday night. It's the night of the week where we have a meal that is simple and not our usual heavy veggie based but we usually still make it at home. Pizza, fish n chips, nachos. And we quite often will have popcorn, homemade banana ice cream or some sweet we don't normally have throughout the week.

For birthdays, Christmas and Easter, we get to have chocolate with our breakfast. These are the only times of the year where we can start our days with something that sweet.

All these little rituals guide our family. They are like our food ship. I know they are special to our kids and I hope that one day, should they have their own families, they will start these rituals for them. When they grow up and leave home, I would like to have a family ritual where together with their own families, we come together once a week or fortnight and we celebrate family over a meal together.

If you want to get some more ideas about the family dinner including fun conversations you can have at the dinner table, check out **the family dinner project (https://thefamilydinnerproject.org/)**. If you have younger kids, a beautiful friend of mine, Mandy dos Santos from Little People Nutrition, has written a book called At The Family Table. It looks at the food on the dinner table of different cultures. It helps children understand the importance of food at the dinner table and that it happens all around the world. You can learn more about the book over at **Little People Nutrition (https://littlepeoplenutrition.com.au/ product/at-my-family-table/)**.

Reduce Stress and Save Yourself Some Time

Yes, it is possible to reduce your stress and save yourself some time (and money) when you eat real food. In The 5 Minute Healthy Lunchbox System eCourse, we help busy parents implement a system that allows them to pack real food lunchboxes, for the whole family, in about five minutes. I share with you below the fundamental rule that underpins this system is the three P's. Planning, Preparation and then Packing or Providing. You can apply these three rules to everything you do food wise at home, not just to lunchboxes. The amount of time you invest in the first two P's has a direct bearing on the amount of time it will take you to pack the lunchboxes or provide the evening meal or snacks.

The first P is for Planning.

This is about working out a rough menu plan for the week. This becomes your road map to keep you on track so even when the wheels are falling off (which we all know they have a tendency to do), you still know what you're doing.

From your menu plan, you create your shopping list. This keeps you on track when you do your shopping. If you know your supermarket well, you can write this list in the order of the aisles, so you know exactly which aisle you need to go into. This also allows you to outsource the task of grocery shopping to your partner or someone who can help you.

It's important to note, planning can be as simple as asking your family what fruits and vegetables they want for the week or it can go further where you discuss what breakfasts, mains, lunches etc they want for the week. I'd suggest providing your family with a few options to choose from rather than just asking hey what do you want. This means you are still making sure you are comfortable with what you want to serve, but they get to take ownership for the choices they make from the options you put forward.

The key to a menu plan is to also think about what you have on during the week. For instance, the weekdays where there is sport, so you get home late or the family eats at different times, you want to plan for food that's quick and simple to provide.

Put your plan up in the kitchen where the family know where it is. This way if they are looking for snacks, they know what's on offer for the week and they know where to find them. We use blue tac and stick ours inside the pantry door.

Do I stay on track with it for every meal? Mostly yes, but sometimes I might go, let's just do a toastie tonight. Stuff happens in the administration of family life. Be kind to yourself but let the plan be your guide too.

The second P is Preparation

Preparation is king or queen to saving your time and stress. Preparation is about carving yourself out a couple of hours during the week to get some of the leg work done for your food. This can be as simple as just washing your produce or it can go a bit further where you wash and pre-cut your fruit and veg to last a few days, or you go the whole hog and cook up some meals and pop them in the fridge or freezer to reheat through the week.

What parents in the eCourse find is that a few weeks of doing prep, allows them to build up a good stash in their freezer so every few weeks there's a prep week that is really light on.

The third P is Pack or Provide

This is really the easiest part. If you have your plan, and you've prepped for the week, then without too much thought you can pack or provide food for your family. Taking the stress out of what to make and how long it takes to make, allows you to put more love into what you're providing your family. Believe it or not, food takes on the energy that we bring to it, and guess what? Those who eat it take on that energy too.

From experience, when our kids have been involved in what's for dinner or what goes into their lunchbox, and I make it calmly and with love, the dinner table is so much more peaceful, and the contents of their lunchbox is more likely to come home eaten. #winning

Create a Cook Club with Friends

Find some like-minded friends who are already feeding their kids real food or who are interested in doing that and join together to have a cook club. Maybe once a fortnight or a month, you all bake a few different things, in big batches, then you share the batch cooking that you've done so every family benefits. For instance, someone may make a big batch of pizza scrolls, someone else some Bolognese sauce, someone else some meatballs, another person some cake. Then agree a date to get together and divide it up between the four of you in the group.

We live in an incredibly blessed world with the internet. We have access to so many recipes at our fingertips. Spend some time googling batch cooking recipes and you'll find thousands. If you want some ideas in one spot, we have loads of free recipes on our website therootcause.com.au.

Find Good Quality Suppliers

This takes a bit of time, but you can save yourself money and buy your family better food if you source your supplies smartly. Some ideas to consider are:

Farmers Markets for Produce

Finding a local Farmers Market serves a few purposes. First, you start to realise what's in season and so shop for what we really should be eating at this time of year. Second, because it's in season, it's cheaper than things which aren't in season that you may buy at the supermarket. Third, you're supporting local growers and they are so grateful for your business, that quite often, they pop a couple of freebies into your bag too. Now that never happens at a supermarket.

There are some other great things about Farmers Markets too. Quite often you will find farmers who offer spray free produce and whilst it's not organic, you are at least minimising your family's exposure to the effects of pesticides. Many Farmers Markets also have tasting plates so if you take your kids along, they get to taste produce and from there, they can choose what appeals to them. You can usually also find a provider of quality meats and truly free range or organic eggs, if you eat these. Oh and incredible bakery breads. Some of the best sourdough breads you can get, you will find at a Farmers Market.

Many Farmers Markets are becoming a great family outing too. Some have entertainment by way of music, jumping castles and activities for the kids. There's usually an awesome local coffee cart and most have great food stalls too. As we travelled Australia, the stand out markets for us were Bulli Showground Farmers Markets, The Greater Whitsunday Food Network Markets, Eumundi Markets and Bellingen Community Markets.

Your Local Butcher or Farmer

If you eat meat, your local butcher is likely to source their meats from local farmers who provides meat to just local clients and stores, rather than big supermarket chains. At least you have a better chance of knowing where your meat comes from. This is important because there won't be lots of food miles and if you do your homework, you can usually find out about the farming practices too.

You may also find a local farmer who is prepared to sell you (and some friends) a whole animal that has been prepared for consumption. Buying in bulk like this can save you a lot of money.

Your Pantry Staples

Today you can take advantage of places who use their power of buying in bulk to provide you with fantastic pantry staples. Flours, grains, nuts, seeds, nut butters, legumes, and more. We love **The Wholefood Collective (https://thewholefoodcollective.com.au/?ref=22)** because we can order it online and we know it has been vetted by our wonderful friend and contributor to this book, Francine Bell, to ensure there are no weird ingredients in them.

Other stores we've used are The Source Bulk Foods, Honest to Goodness, and we also love our local store Whole n Happy in Gladstone on the Mid North Coast of NSW.

Being A Stand for Children's Health

I've left this to last because it's so important. If we want our children and their friends, and kids generally, to reach their full potential, then it is going to take us parents to be a stand for their health.

This means we need to be prepared to go into bat for them. To ensure our voice is counted. You can show you are serious about children's health by:

1. Vote with your shopping dollar

The only way manufacturers will stop making processed food that is not the best for our children's health, is if enough of us stop buying it. Every time you buy a processed food, it sends a message to the supermarkets and the manufacturers the product is needed. Ask yourself is it really necessary? Can you buy something better? Do you need to buy it? Make your child's health matter by using your shopping dollars wisely.

2. Push for food education in our schools

Kids just want to fit in. You probably already realise what their friends eat has a big bearing on what your kids want to eat too. At school there is a lot of focus on physical activity but not as much on nutrition. We need children, parents and teachers to understand the connection between what they are eating and the impacts it is having on health and academic results. Food is literally having an impact on the potential of our kids to fulfil on their future.

We invite you to stand with us for Children's Health, and talk to the decision makers at your school about food education.

Teaching kids to cook and grow food is important and there are some great education programs out there specifically for this. Jamie Oliver's Learn Your Fruit and Vegetables Program and Stephanie Alexander's Kitchen Garden Program are probably two of the higher profile programs. Both are excellent programs. It would be beneficial to reinstate the good old Home Economics class as a permanent curriculum item too.

The food education The Root Cause provides focuses on empowering students, teachers and parents with knowledge of **why** it's important to make better food choices for their body and providing them with the tools and life skills necessary to navigate today's processed food world.

Our Children's Health Program is a partnership program for schools. At the heart of the Children's Health Program is our well known and impactful Mad Food Science Incursion. Schools can partner with us in two ways:

1. **Short Term Focus** – this includes The Mad Food Science Incursion for students (and teachers learn from this too), the Parent Seminar and A Food and Waste Report to provide the school with important data.

2. **Longer Term Focus** – this is where we partner with individual schools for an entire year or more. The goal is to create lasting change in the way students, teachers, and parents think about – and make choices around – food and sleep. It includes The Mad Food Science Incursion, the Parent Seminar, the Food and Waste Report, a Teacher Professional Development course, a FREE yearly online membership for parents to our Parent Portal with a host of resources to support parents and children at home, plus ongoing support for the school.

We want to partner with schools who want to be leaders in student and teacher wellbeing.

Simple Steps To Bring Our Work To Your School
- **Visit our website** and submit your schools details
  http://rootcau.se/cometomyschool
- **One of our Certified Instructors** will contact you and your school

- **Find Supporters** (fellow parents, teachers, P&C/F members etc) at your school who are all advocates for eating more real food, and get them to support your plan to bring our work to your school.
- **Share your passion** with the decision makers at the school. Book an appointment to see the Principal or other appropriate decision maker and share your passion for our work, including the support you have for bringing The Children's Health Program to your school.
- **Follow Up and be persistent!** Please remember, following up with people is not nagging, it's about being of service. The truth is school decision makers are busy people, so think of following them up in the same way as an SMS reminder service you get when you book a dental or doctor's appointment – it's a helpful, gentle reminder.

3. Be Prepared to Swim in the Opposite Direction

It has taken us thirty years to get to the point where most people feel processed foods are normal, so it's not like we can flick a switch tomorrow and it will change people's behaviour. Being a stand for children's health is going to require you to be prepared to swim in the opposite direction to many of your family and friends. But do so unashamedly. What you role-model to your kids at home about the way you eat, is likely to become what they turn to as the way they eat when they leave home. The way you eat at home, is likely to impact your child in so many ways during their growing and learning years, but also as they become adults.

Long-term health effects are a result of many short term food choices. Thank you for Standing For Children's Health!

PART 4:

Appendices
&
Reference

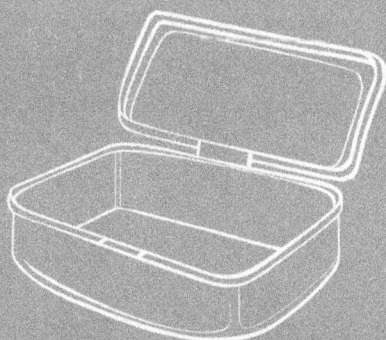

Appendix 1
Lunchbox Product Reference

A More Detailed Look at "What's In My Food?"

The information in this appendix takes a closer look at the individual products within the product categories that we reviewed. Due to the number of products we have reviewed, it is not feasible to show all nutrition information for each product. We have included enough information for you at a quick glance to think about whether you want to take a closer look at this product or find an alternate one. If you want to go to the next level of data, we have created an Online Product Companion.

Our Intention for You

The intention of this information is for you to find the product and brand you shop for and learn what's in the food. From there you can make a choice about whether you wish to continue including it as a lunchbox food for your child(ren) or whether you will find a better choice or even find a recipe to make it at home.

It is not intended this information be used for a comparison across the brands within category. The contributors in this book will not be drawn into discussion about comparing products within brand. This book is merely designed to raise awareness about the importance of lunchbox food and what's in common lunchbox packet foods. We strongly encourage you to use the information in the previous chapters and this one, to make better and more conscious choices for your family.

With all this information you have available, you can now make the following choices:

For each specific packet food:
- Keep buying the product if you decide it's OK for your child
- Find a replacement packet food that is better for your child
- Find a recipe and make a healthier alternative at home
- Eliminate the packet food altogether

You can then decide how often your child gets to eat the packet food:
- Every day in the school lunchbox
- Only "sometimes" in the school lunchbox
- Only "sometimes" at home
- Not at all

As you'll see from the data, most packet foods are best left out of school lunchboxes, and minimised overall in the best interests of our children's health.

Remember, the easiest, healthiest and cheapest replacement for packet foods is fruit and vegetables.

Important notes:

1. Food manufacturers do from time to time reformulate their products. The information in this book was prepared on the foods on the supermarket shelf between December 2018 and February 2019.

2. The Detailed Information is shown for the per serve amount, not per 100g. For most packet foods a serve is what your kids will be consuming, so you need to know what is in the serve.

3. In the table below, a Yes in the column Contains Additives and Potential Effects means the product contains an additive identified in the Chemical Maze as having potential effects that could impact different elements of a child's health. Please remember, this is about awareness. You may think your child is not affected by additives and preservatives, but until you remove foods including these for a while, how do you really know if your child is affected? The Online Product Companion lists details of the additives and their potential effects.

You can order the Online Product Companion at
http://thelunchboxeffect.com/opc

The products in this Appendix are grouped in order of how common they are in lunchboxes:

- Chips - p240
- Muesli & Other Bars - p252
- Savoury Crackers - p264
- Sweet Biscuits - p271
- Juice & Flavoured Milks - p276
- Yoghurt Tubs & Pouches - p284
- Chocolate & Lollies - p295
- Fruit & Jelly Cups - p298
- Bread & Wraps - p300

Chips

Product Name	No. of Ingredients	Sugar (g)	Sugar (tsp)	Sugar in Top 3?	Sodium (mg)	Fat (g)	No. of Additives	Additives have potential effects?
Ajitas Vege Chips Chicken Style	17	1.9	0.5	No	252	3.9	1	Yes
Ajitas Vege Chips Snack BBQ	14	1.7	0.4	No	151	4	1	
Ajitas Vege Chips Snack Natural	7	1.5	0.4	No	118	3.9	0.0	
Ajitas Vege Chips Snack Sea Salt and Vinegar	11	2.5	0.6	No	225	3.7	2	
Ajitas Vege Twists Cheese Max	17	0.1	0.0	No	216	2.9	3	Yes
Blackstone Caramel Popcorn	9	5.3	1.3	Yes	53	3.3	2	
Blackstone Deli Style Potato Chips Honey Soy Chicken	19	1.1	0.3	Yes	102	7.8	7	Yes
Blackstone Deli Style Potato Chips Sea Salt	3	0.1	0.0	No	155	8.2	0.0	

Product Name	No. of Ingredients	Sugar (g)	Sugar (tsp)	Sugar in Top 3?	Sodium (mg)	Fat (g)	No. of Additives	Additives have potential effects?
Blackstone Deli Style Potato Chips Sea Salt and Balsamic Vinegar	11	0.5	0.1	No	216	7.9	4	Yes
Blackstone Deli Style Potato Chips Sweet Chilli and Sour Cream	12	0.8	0.2	Yes	159	7.9	4	Yes
Blackstone Sweet and Salty Popcorn	4	2.5	0.6	Yes	58	3.3	0.0	
Chazoos Noodle Snak BBQ Flavour	16	0.5	0.1	No	138	5.6	6	Yes
Chazoos Noodle Snak Chicken Flavour	17	0.4	0.1	No	188	5.8	5	Yes
Chazoos Salted Popcorn Multi Pack	3	<1	0.0	No	137	5.2	0.0	
Cheetos Cheese & Bacon Balls	13	0.7	0.2	No	120	5.5	4	Yes
Cobs Natural Popcorn Cheddar Cheese	10	0.4	0.1	No	72	3.2	2	

Product Name	No. of Ingredients	Sugar (g)	Sugar (tsp)	Sugar in Top 3?	Sodium (mg)	Fat (g)	No. of Additives	Additives have potential effects?
Cobs Natural Popcorn Lightly Salted, Slightly Sweet	4	2.1	0.5	Yes	35	2.9	0.0	
Cobs Natural Popcorn Sea Salt	3	0.1	0.0	No	47	3.2	0.0	
Coles Deli Style Potato Chips Multipack Honey Soy Chicken	16	<1	0.0	Yes	71	4.7	2	
Coles Deli Style Potato Chips Multipack Natural Sea Salt	3	<1	0.0	No	81	4.8	0.0	
Coles Deli Style Potato Chips Multipack Sea Salt & Balsamic Vinegar	12	<1	0.0	No	146	4.9	5	Yes
Coles Noodle Snacks Chicken Flavour	15	0.1	0.0	No	191	4.3	4	Yes
Coles Original Crinkle Cut Chips	3	<1	0.0	No	104	6.5	0.0	
Coles Original Popcorn	3	0.1	0.0	No	114	5.3	0.0	

Product Name	No. of Ingredients	Sugar (g)	Sugar (tsp)	Sugar in Top 3?	Sodium (mg)	Fat (g)	No. of Additives	Additives have potential effects?
Cool Pak Popcorn	3	0.0	0.0	No	138	5.2	0.0	
Doritos Cheese Supreme	23	0.4	0.1	No	117	5.1	8	Yes
Freedom Foods Messy Monkeys Burger Flavour	14	0.2	0.1	No	79	3.6	1	
French Fries Original Crunchy Potato Straws	3	0.5	0.1	No	133	6.2	0.0	
Grain Waves Sour Cream & Chives	18	1.5	0.4	No	85	4.9	6	
Harvest Snaps Baked Pea Crisps Original	14	0.5	0.1	No	72	3.7	4	Yes
Harvest Snaps Baked Pea Crisps Salt & Vinegar	15	0.4	0.1	No	132	3.7	7	Yes
Healtheriers Kidscare Potato Curls Chicken Flavour	25	<1mg	0.0	No	71	1.1	10	Yes

Product Name	No. of Ingredients	Sugar (g)	Sugar (tsp)	Sugar in Top 3?	Sodium (mg)	Fat (g)	No. of Additives	Additives have potential effects?
Healtheriers Kidscare Potato Stix Chicken	16	<1mg	0.0	No	131	2.7	4	
Healtheriers Kidscare Potato Stix Roast Potato	16	<1mg	0.0	No	116	2.7	5	
Healtheriers Kidscare Rice Wheels Burger	19	0.4	0.1	Yes	91	1.7	6	
Healtheriers Kidscare Rice Wheels Cheese	15	0.6	0.2	No	127	1.8	4	
Healtheriers Kidscare Rice Wheels Roast Chicken	17	0.3	0.1	Yes	131	1.4	5	
J.J. Snacks Chicken Flavour	12	1.4	0.4	No	135	3.4	3	Yes
Jumpy's Chicken Flavour	18	0.3	0.1	No	154	5.9	5	Yes
Jumpy's Original Flavour	10	0.8	0.2	No	136	5.9	3	Yes

Product Name	No. of Ingredients	Sugar (g)	Sugar (tsp)	Sugar in Top 3?	Sodium (mg)	Fat (g)	No. of Additives	Additives have potential effects?
Jumpy's Salt & Vinegar Flavour	11	0.1	0.0	No	227	5.9	4	Yes
Kettle MultiPack Chips Honey Soy Chicken	12	0.6	0.2	Yes	95	4.8	2	Yes
Kettle MultiPack Chips Salt & Vingegar	11	0.3	0.1	Yes	149	4.7	4	Yes
Kettle MultiPack Chips Sea Salt	3	0.0	0.0	No	90	5	0.0	
Macro Quinoa Puffs Cheesy Flavour	16	<1	0.0	No	71	<1	2	Yes
Macro Quinoa Puffs Chicken Flavour	16	<1	0.0	No	71	<1	2	
Mamee Monster Noodle Snack Bbq Flavour	16	0.5	0.1	No	199	5.6	5	Yes
Mamee Monster Noodle Snack Chicken Flavour	19	0.4	0.1	No	188	5.8	4	Yes

Product Name	No. of Ingredients	Sugar (g)	Sugar (tsp)	Sugar in Top 3?	Sodium (mg)	Fat (g)	No. of Additives	Additives have potential effects?
Messy Monkeys Salted Popcorn	3	0.1	0.0	No	46	2.8	0.0	
Messy Monkeys Sweet & Salty Popcorn	4	1	0.3	Yes	31	2.6	0.0	
Messy Monkeys Wholegrain Bites Cheese	11	0.1	0.0	No	80	3.6	1	
Messy Monkeys Wholegrain Bites Chicken	14	0.6	0.2	No	89	3.7	1	
Parkers Original Preztels	4	2.7	0.7	Yes	140	2.1	0.0	
Pringles Minis Chicken	19	0.3	0.075	No	134	5.4	7	Yes
Pringles Minis Original	24	0.4	0.1	No	140	5.4	8	Yes
Pringles Minis Sour Cream & Onion	23	0.4	0.1	No	140	5.4	8	Yes

Product Name	No. of Ingredients	Sugar (g)	Sugar (tsp)	Sugar in Top 3?	Sodium (mg)	Fat (g)	No. of Additives	Additives have potential effects?
Red Rock Deli Deli Style Potato Chips Honey Soy Chicken	20	1.5	0.4	Yes	146	6.6	3	Yes
Red Rock Deli Deli Style Potato Chips Sea Salt	3	0.3	0.1	No	140	6.4	0.0	
Red Rock Deli Deli Style Potato Chips Seat Salt & Balsamic Vinegar	13	0.7	0.2	No	205	6.7	4	Yes
Red Rock Deli Deli Style Potato Chips Sweet Chilli & Sour Cream	22	1.5	0.4	Yes	192	6.5	6	Yes
Sakata Rice Crisps Honey Soy	16	0.9	0.2	Yes	92	5.3	3	
Smiths 20 Pack Barbeque Flavoured Chips	19	0.6	0.15	No	94	6.3	8	Yes
Smiths 20 Pack Chicken Flavoured Chips	19	0.5	0.125	No	95	6.3	8	Yes
Smiths 20 Pack Original Chips	8	0.2	0.05	No	106	6.6	4	Yes

Product Name	No. of Ingredients	Sugar (g)	Sugar (tsp)	Sugar in Top 3?	Sodium (mg)	Fat (g)	No. of Additives	Additives have potential effects?
Smiths 20 Pack Salt & Vinegar Flavoured Chips	15	0.6	0.15	No	151	6.3	7	Yes
Smiths Fun Mix 20 Pack Burger Rings	19	0.5	0.1	No	172	5	9	Yes
Smiths Fun Mix 20 Pack Cheese Flavoured Twisties	19	1.1	0.3	No	172	4.4	8	Yes
Smiths Fun Mix 20 Pack Cheeto Cheese & Bacon Flavour	13	0.7	0.2	No	120	5.5	4	Yes
Smiths Fun Mix 20 Pack Original	8	0.2	0.1	No	106	6.6	3	
Smiths Fun Mix 20 Pack Salt & Vinegar	15	0.6	0.2	No	151	6.3	6	Yes
Sprinters Crinkle Cut MultiPack Chips Barbeque	17	0.7	0.2	Yes	119	6.4	5	Yes
Sprinters Crinkle Cut MultiPack Chips Chicken	16	0.5	0.1	Yes	123	6.4	5	

Product Name	No. of Ingredients	Sugar (g)	Sugar (tsp)	Sugar in Top 3?	Sodium (mg)	Fat (g)	No. of Additives	Additives have potential effects?
Sprinters Crinkle Cut MultiPack Chips Original	3	0.1	0.0	No	122	6.8	0.0	
Sprinters Crinkle Cut MultiPack Chips Salt & Vinegar	11	0.2	0.1	No	217	6.4	4	
Sprinters Elotra Cheese Flavoured Corn Chips	19	0.5	0.1	Yes	107	5.1	6	Yes
Sunbites Air Popped Popcorn Lightly Salted	3	0.0	0.0	No	64	2.8	0.0	
The Natural Chip Co. Sea salt	3	0.1	0.0	No	161	8.9	0.0	
Top 20 Family Favourites MultiPack CC's Tasty Cheese	18	0.6	0.2	No	169	4.8	7	Yes
Top 20 Family Favourites MultiPack Cheezels Original Cheese	16	0.9	0.2	No	228	6.5	5	Yes
Top 20 Family Favourites MultiPack French Fries	3	0.6	0.2	No	133	6.2	0.0	

Product Name	No. of Ingredients	Sugar (g)	Sugar (tsp)	Sugar in Top 3?	Sodium (mg)	Fat (g)	No. of Additives	Additives have potential effects?
Top 20 Family Favourites MultiPack Honey Soy Chicken	13	0.5	0.1	Yes	134	6.4	2	
Top 20 Family Favourites MultiPack Light & Tangy	14	0.8	0.2	Yes	132	5.9	4	Yes
Top 20 Family Favourites MultiPack Thins Original	3	0.5	0.1	No	108	6.2	0.0	
Twisties Chicken Flavour	17	0.5	0.1	No	150	5.2	5	Yes
Woolworths Chees Twists	16	0.4	0.1	No	180	4.3	6	Yes
Woolworths MultiPack Cheese Flavoured Rings	18	0.4	0.1	No	184	5.4	6	Yes
Woolworths MultiPack Crink Cut Original	3	0.1	0.0	No	98	7.3	0.0	
Woolworths MultiPack Salt & Vinegar Flavoured Crink Cut	11	0.1	0.0	No	201	6.4	5	

Product Name	No. of Ingredients	Sugar (g)	Sugar (tsp)	Sugar in Top 3?	Sodium (mg)	Fat (g)	No. of Additives	Additives have potential effects?
Woolworths MultiPack Supreme Cheese Flavoured	20	0.3	0.1	Yes	95	4.4	6	Yes
Woolworths Origianl Popcorn	3	0.7	0.2	No	77	5.1	0.0	
Woolworths Original Crinkle Cut	3	0.1	0.0	No	98	7.3	0.0	

Muesli & Other Bars

Product Name	No. of Ingredients	Sugar (g)	Sugar (tsp)	Sugar in Top 3?	Sodium (mg)	Fat (g)	No. of Additives	Additives have potential effects?
Bear Real Fruit Yo Yos Mango	3	8.4	2.1	No	<5	<1	0.0	
Cadbury Milk Chocolate Cake Bars	33	8.3	2.1	Yes	59	4.8	6	Yes
Cadbury Mini Rolls Milk Chocolate	32	9.8	2.5	Yes	64	5.3	10	Yes
Cadbury Mini Rolls Raspberry	40	11.8	3.0	Yes	58	5.1	14	Yes
Carman's Classic Fruit & Nut Muesli Bars	17	7.8	1.95	No	9	6.7	1	
Carman's Dark Choc Blueberry Superfood Bars	22	8.1	2.0	Yes	4	6.6	2	
Carman's Dark Choc Cranberry & Almond Bars	23	8.4	2.1	Yes	6	5.8	3	
Carman's Greek Style Yoghurt Fruit & Nut Bars	22	7.3	1.825	Yes	6	6.1	4	Yes

Product Name	No. of Ingredients	Sugar (g)	Sugar (tsp)	Sugar in Top 3?	Sodium (mg)	Fat (g)	No. of Additives	Additives have potential effects?
Carman's Oat Slice Bites Belgian Chocolate Brownie	17	5.9	1.5	No	31	4.8	3	
Carman's Oat Slice Bites Golden Oat & Coconut	11	4.7	1.2	No	35	5.2	1	
Carman's Original Fruit Free Muesli Bars	12	5.4	1.4	No	6	9	1	
Carman's Super Berry Muesli Bars	17	6.8	1.7	No	11	8.6	1	
Coles Chewy Bars Milk Choc	18	6.2	1.6	Yes	12	3.8	6	Yes
Coles Choc Chip Muesli Bars	17	6.5	1.6	Yes	<5	3.2	4	Yes
Coles Fruit Filled Bars Apple & Cinnamon	20	13.7	3.4	No	62	<1	4	Yes
Coles Fruit Filled Bars Apricot Flavour	23	12.7	3.2	No	63	<1	8	Yes

Product Name	No. of Ingredients	Sugar (g)	Sugar (tsp)	Sugar in Top 3?	Sodium (mg)	Fat (g)	No. of Additives	Additives have potential effects?
Coles Fruit Filled Bars Mixed Berry	23	15	3.8	No	60	<1	5	Yes
Coles Fruit Sticks	22	14.2	3.6	Yes	12	<1	5	Yes
Coles Fruitops Passion-fruit Bars	23	7.8	2.0	Yes	24	3.4	7	Yes
Coles Fruitops Strawber-ry Bars	25	7.4	1.9	Yes	27	3.5	8	Yes
Coles Strawberry Yoghurt Topped Muesli Bars	17	7.7	1.9	Yes	7	3.7	4	Yes
Coles Yoghurt Bars Strawberry	20	7.4	1.9	Yes	11	3.8	5	Yes
Freedom Messy Monkey Snack Bars Apple Pie	17	5.7	1.4	No	17	1	4	
Freedom Messy Monkeys Snack Bars Mango & Apple	8	6.7	1.7	No	6	1.7	0.0	

Product Name	No. of Ingredients	Sugar (g)	Sugar (tsp)	Sugar in Top 3?	Sodium (mg)	Fat (g)	No. of Additives	Additives have potential effects?
Freedom Messy Monkeys Strawberry & Apple	8	6.7	1.7	No	7	1.8	0.0	
Hillcrest Bubble Bars Choc Chip	25	5.4	1.4	Yes	35	1.5	10	Yes
Hillcrest Bubble Bars Choc Rainbow Rice Crispy Bars	37	5.3	1.3	Yes	33	1.5	15	Yes
Hillcrest Caramel Muffin Bars	36	9.8	2.5	Yes	208	3.8	18	Yes
Hillcrest Chewy Choc Muesli Bars	26	4.8	1.2	Yes	23	5.3	10	Yes
Hillcrest Chewy Yoghurt Muesli Bars Apricot & Yoghurt	33	9.7	2.4	Yes	40	4.7	11	Yes
Hillcrest Chewy Yoghurt Muesli Bars Strawberry	37	5.5	1.4	Yes	9	4.9	17	Yes
Hillcrest Chewy Yoghurt Muesli Bars Strawberry & Yoghurt	39	8.7	2.2	Yes	23	5.3	16	Yes

Product Name	No. of Ingredients	Sugar (g)	Sugar (tsp)	Sugar in Top 3?	Sodium (mg)	Fat (g)	No. of Additives	Additives have potential effects?
Hillcrest Chewy Yoghurt Muesli Bars Tropical & Yoghurt	36	8.8	2.2	Yes	25	5.4	13	Yes
Hillcrest Choc Chip Coconut Protein Oat Bars	27	10.4	2.6	Yes	88	10.4	12	Yes
Hillcrest Choc Fudge Muffin Bars	36	10.4	2.6	Yes	191	4.2	18	Yes
Hillcrest Crunchtop Muesli Bars Raspberry	28	8.8	2.2	Yes	29	3.7	6	Yes
Hillcrest Dark Chocolate Protein Oat Bars	24	11.3	2.8	Yes	100	9.7	11	Yes
Hillcrest Fruit & Nut Muesli Bars	17	7.6	1.9	Yes	10	7.9	2	
Hillcrest Fruity Filled Bars Apple & Cinnamon	24	11.9	3.0	No	81	1.2	11	Yes
Hillcrest Fruity Filled Bars Blueberry	25	11.2	2.8	No	81	1.2	11	Yes

Product Name	No. of Ingredients	Sugar (g)	Sugar (tsp)	Sugar in Top 3?	Sodium (mg)	Fat (g)	No. of Additives	Additives have potential effects?
Hillcrest Fruity Filled Bars Mixed Berry	28	11.7	2.9	No	81	1.2	12	Yes
Hillcrest Milk Chocolate Rice Cake Bars	6	5.5	1.4	Yes	14	4.5	1	
Hillcrest Morning Break Chocolate	33	8	2.0	Yes	58	2	15	Yes
Hillcrest Morning Break Strawberry	36	8.5	2.1	Yes	58	1.8	15	Yes
Hillcrest Oat Bars Choc Chip	27	14.6	3.7	Yes	82	9.4	12	Yes
Hillcrest Oat Bars Golden Oats	16	8.7	2.2	No	91	10	8	Yes
Hillcrest Peanut Butter Protein Oat Bars	26	9.8	2.45	Yes	179	11.7	10	
Hillcrest Strawberry Flavoured Rice Cake Bars	7	5.5	1.4	Yes	14	4.5	2	

Product Name	No. of Ingredients	Sugar (g)	Sugar (tsp)	Sugar in Top 3?	Sodium (mg)	Fat (g)	No. of Additives	Additives have potential effects?
Hillcrest Triple Berry Muesli Bars	28	8.1	2.025	Yes	9	7.7	6	Yes
Kellogg's Special Biscuit Moments Chocolate Flavour	35	6.9	1.7	Yes	68	2.5	16	Yes
LCMs Choc Chip	28	6.9	1.7	Yes	56	2.2	11	Yes
LCMs Cocopops	28	8.5	2.1	Yes	39	3	10	Yes
LCMs Kaleidos	37	7.6	1.9	Yes	50	2.1	16	Yes
LCMs Splitstix Banana Choc	28	8.8	2.2	Yes	54	3.4	11	Yes
LCMs Splitstix Choco-latey	30	7.5	1.9	Yes	46	2.8	10	Yes
LCMs Splitstix Yoghurty	27	7.9	2.0	Yes	51	3.2	9	Yes

Product Name	No. of Ingredients	Sugar (g)	Sugar (tsp)	Sugar in Top 3?	Sodium (mg)	Fat (g)	No. of Additives	Additives have potential effects?
Mother Earth Baked Oaty Slices Chocolate Oats	29	10.9	2.7	No	107	7.7	5	
Mother Earth Baked Oaty Slices Very Berry	29	11.4	2.9	Yes	104	5.3	6	Yes
Nature Valley Crunch Canadian Maple Syrup	10	11.6	2.9	Yes	112	7.4	3	
Nature Valley Crunch Oats & Dark Chocolate	14	11.7	2.9	Yes	98	8.3	3	
Nature Valley Crunch Oats & Honey	8	11.7	2.9	Yes	123	7.5	2	
Nestle Milo Dipped Snack Bars with White Chocolate	37	6.5	1.6	Yes	27	2.6	10	Yes
Nestle Milo Snack Bars Original	33	4.6	1.2	Yes	23	1.1	8	Yes
Nice&Natural Protein Wholeseed Bars Cranberry & Raspberry	17	3.2	0.8	Yes	54	8.7	5	Yes

Product Name	No. of Ingredients	Sugar (g)	Sugar (tsp)	Sugar in Top 3?	Sodium (mg)	Fat (g)	No. of Additives	Additives have potential effects?
NRG Maxx Snack Bar Original	34	5.1	1.3	No	20	1	15	Yes
NRG Maxx Snack Bar with Milk	40	7.2	1.8	No	25	2.8	16	Yes
Nutri-grain Choc	29	8.5	2.1	No	60	2.4	8	Yes
Nutri-grain Original	29	8.7	2.2	No	51	2.3	8	Yes
Roll-ups Fun Prints Strawberry	20	4.2	1.1	Yes	8	0.5	10	Yes
Roll-ups Rainbow Berry berry	20	4.2	1.1	Yes	8	0.5	10	Yes
Roll-ups Rainbow Fruit Salad	20	4.1	1.0	Yes	8	0.5	8	Yes
Scooby-Doo! Iddy Biddy Fruit Bits	17	11.9	3.0	No	8	0.2	6	Yes
Skadoos	18	10.4	2.6	Yes	28	4.6	7	Yes

Product Name	No. of Ingredients	Sugar (g)	Sugar (tsp)	Sugar in Top 3?	Sodium (mg)	Fat (g)	No. of Additives	Additives have potential effects?
The Cake Stall Cake Bars Chocolate Chip	26	13.1	3.3	Yes	118	8	12	Yes
The Cake Stall Mini Muffins 3x Double Choc Chip & 3x Blueberry	30	10.3	2.6	Yes	104	8.6	18	Yes
Uncle Toby's Chewy Lamington Flavour	22	4.3	1.1	Yes	7	3.4	6	Yes
Uncle Toby's Lunchbox Favourites Chewy Choc Chip	28	5.4	1.4	Yes	13	3.6	7	Yes
Uncle Toby's Lunchbox Favourites Chewy Forest Fruits	24	5.4	1.4	Yes	4	2.8	6	Yes
Uncle Toby's Lunchbox Favourites Yoghurt Strawberry	29	5.8	1.5	Yes	6	3.5	9	Yes
Uncle Toby's Milk & Oats Vanilla Flavour	21	6.2	1.6	Yes	47	4.4	9	Yes
Uncle Toby's Yoghurt Honeycomb Flavour	32	5.2	1.3	Yes	6	3.8	13	

Product Name	No. of Ingredients	Sugar (g)	Sugar (tsp)	Sugar in Top 3?	Sodium (mg)	Fat (g)	No. of Additives	Additives have potential effects?
Uncle Toby's Yoghurt Mango Passionfruit	29	5.7	1.4	Yes	7	3.5	11	
Uncle Toby's Yoghurt Strawberry Flavour	29	5.8	1.5	Yes	6	3.5	9	
Woolworths Banana Muffin Bars	24	11.8	3.0	Yes	137	6.7	13	Yes
Woolworths Chewy Muesli Bars Choc Drizzle	17	5	1.3	Yes	20	3	4	Yes
Woolworths Chewy Muesli Bars Honeycomb	26	5.9	1.5	Yes	20	3.2	5	Yes
Woolworths Double Choc Muffin Bars	28	12.5	3.1	Yes	129	7.7	13	Yes
Woolworths Fruit Filled Bars Apple Flavoured	21	10.4	2.6	Yes	56	<1	6	Yes
Woolworths Muesli Bars Choc Chip	15	6.6	1.7	Yes	<5	3.3	5	Yes

Product Name	No. of Ingredients	Sugar (g)	Sugar (tsp)	Sugar in Top 3?	Sodium (mg)	Fat (g)	No. of Additives	Additives have potential effects?
Woolworths Muesli Bars Yoghurt & Strawberry Flavour	28	7.1	1.8	Yes	6	3.3	8	Yes
Woolworths Oven Baked Fruit Filled Bars Apple & Blueberry Flavoured	21	10.9	2.7	Yes	52	<1	5	Yes
Woolworths Yoghurt Muesli Bars Apricot	20	5.2	1.3	Yes	10	3.1	5	Yes

Savoury Crackers

Product Name	No. of Ingredients	Sugar (g)	Sugar (tsp)	Sugar in Top 3?	Sodium (mg)	Fat (g)	No. of Additives	Additives have potential effects?
Arnott's Minis JATZ Original	11	1.3	0.3	Yes	138	4.4	3	
Arnott's Shapes Barbeque Flavour	21	0.2	0.1	No	171	5.6	6	Yes
Arnott's Shapes Light & Crispy Balsamic Vinegar & Sea Salt	22	0.6	0.2	No	178	2.9	9	Yes
Arnott's Shapes Light & Crispy Sour Cream & Chives	23	0.6	0.2	No	154	2.9	9	Yes
Arnott's Shapes Light & Crispy Tasty Cheddar & Chives	26	0.5	0.1	No	170	2.9	11	Yes
Arnott's Shapes Mini Crimpy Chicken Flavour	17	1.7	0.4	Yes	216	4.9	8	Yes
Arnott's Shapes Pizza Flavour	25	0.4	0.1	No	155	5.8	7	
Arnott's Tiny Teddy Cheesy Crackers	18	0.8	0.2	No	83	4.4	5	

Product Name	No. of Ingredients	Sugar (g)	Sugar (tsp)	Sugar in Top 3?	Sodium (mg)	Fat (g)	No. of Additives	Additives have potential effects?
Bega Farmers' Tasty Sticks	4	<1	0.0	No	144	7.1	0.0	
Bega Stringers Original	4	<1	0.0	No	130	4.5	0.0	
Bega Stringers Tasty Cheddar Cheese Flavour	5	<1	0.0	No	130	4.5	1	
Coles Cheddar Cheese Snack Packs	29	1.2	0.3	No	198	5.8	10	Yes
Coles French Onion Flavoured Snack Packs	29	1.2	0.3	No	189	5.5	10	Yes
Coles Snack Packs Cheese Spread & Crispbread	45	<1	0.0	No	290	5.6	15	Yes
Cowbelle Cheese Triangles Spreadable Processed Cheese	11	1.1	0.3	No	175	4.7	4	Yes
Cowbelle Cheese Triangles Spreadable Processed Cheese Light	12	1.1	0.3	No	175	1.7	6	Yes

Product Name	No. of Ingredients	Sugar (g)	Sugar (tsp)	Sugar in Top 3?	Sodium (mg)	Fat (g)	No. of Additives	Additives have potential effects?
Dairyworks Colby Natural Cheese & Rice Crackers	7	<1	0.0	No	190	8.8	0.0	
Damora Barbeque Snakos	14	0.6	0.2	No	249	4.9	6	Yes
Damora Bbq Flavour Rice Crackers	16	1	0.3	Yes	147	1.4	5	Yes
Damora Cheese Flavour Rice Crackers	24	0.6	0.2	No	184	1.7	7	Yes
Damora Dippits Cheddar Cheese Spread & Crispbread	29	1.2	0.3	No	198	5.8	10	Yes
Damora Dippits French Onion Cheese Spread & Crispbread	30	1.2	0.3	No	189	5.5	10	Yes
Damora Dippits Tasty Cheese Spread & Crispbread	30	1.6	0.4	No	206	5.3	10	Yes
Damora ETON Original Cracker Biscuits	10	1	0.3	No	66	2.7	3	

Product Name	No. of Ingredients	Sugar (g)	Sugar (tsp)	Sugar in Top 3?	Sodium (mg)	Fat (g)	No. of Additives	Additives have potential effects?
Damora Mini Brown Rice Cakes Cheese Flavoured	12	1	0.3	No	122	2.2	4	
Damora Mini Brown Rice Cakes Chicken Flavoured	14	0.3	0.1	Yes	108	2.2	4	
Damora Mini Brown Rice Cakes Original Flavoured	3	0.2	0.1	No	104	2.2	0.0	
Damora Original Rice Crackers	4	0.1	0.0	No	97	0.7	0.0	
Damora Pizza Snakos	15	0.8	0.2	No	174	5.3	4	
Damora Seaweed Rice Crackers	8	1.4	0.4	No	249	0.3	0.0	
Damora Thin & Crispy Rice Crackers Original	10	0.1	0.0	Yes	66	1.5	4	Yes
Damora Thin & Crispy Rice Crackers Salt & Vinegar	9	0.1	0.0	Yes	138	1.5	5	Yes

Product Name	No. of Ingredients	Sugar (g)	Sugar (tsp)	Sugar in Top 3?	Sodium (mg)	Fat (g)	No. of Additives	Additives have potential effects?
Damora Topz Crackers Original	9	1.4	0.4	No	202	3.5	4	
Homebrand Cheese Dip & Crispbread Cheddar Cheese Flavour	45	1.4	0.4	No	275	6.1	18	Yes
Homebrand Cheese Dip & Crispbread French Onion Flavour	47	1.4	0.4	No	275	6.1	19	Yes
Mainland Cheese & Crackers On The Go Tasty	16	<1	0.0	No	188	7.9	3	
Mainland Munchables Tasty Cheese & Crackers	24	<1	0.0	No	248	8.5	7	Yes
Peckish Salt & Vinegar Flavoured Rice Crackers	8	<0.1	0.0	Yes	140	1.3	1	
Peckish Sour Cream & Chive Flavoured Rice Crackers	10	0.3	0.1	No	104	1.5	2	
Peckish Tangy Bbq Flavoured Rice Crackers	8	0.9	0.2	Yes	102	1.2	1	

Product Name	No. of Ingredients	Sugar (g)	Sugar (tsp)	Sugar in Top 3?	Sodium (mg)	Fat (g)	No. of Additives	Additives have potential effects?
Ritz Mini Original	13	2.1	0.5	Yes	130	5.7	6	
Sakata Authentic Rice Crackers Seaweed	12	1.2	0.3	No	243	0.3	1	
Sakata Wholegrain Authentic Rice Crackers Original	8	0.4	0.1	No	99	2	0.0	
SunBites Snack Crackers with Quinoa Cheddar & Chives	16	1.3	0.3	No	73	5.4	2	
SunRice Rice Cake Bites Sea Salt & Rosemary Flavour	11	<1	0.0	Yes	265	4.4	1	
SunRice Rice Cake Bites Sour Cream & Chives Flavour	18	<1	0.0	No	215	5.2	4	Yes
Uncle Toby's LeSnack Cheddar Cheese Flavour	30	1.1	0.3	No	185	5.5	10	Yes
Uncle Toby's LeSnack French Onion Flavour	32	1.1	0.3	No	175	5.3	10	Yes

Product Name	No. of Ingredients	Sugar (g)	Sugar (tsp)	Sugar in Top 3?	Sodium (mg)	Fat (g)	No. of Additives	Additives have potential effects?
Uncle Toby's LeSnack Tasty Cheese Flavour	33	1.5	0.4	No	195	5.1	10	Yes
Westacre Snack'N'Go Kids Colby Cheese with Rice Crackers	15	0.3	0.1	No	151	7	3	Yes
Westacre Snack'N'Go Tasty Cheddar Cheese with Water Crackers	9	0.2	0.1	No	182	8	2	
Woolworths Cheese Thin Rice Crackers Minis	11	<1	0.0	No	48	2.7	4	
Woolworths Light Tasty Cheese & Crackers	16	<0.5	0.0	No	188	6	3	
Woolworths Natural Cheese Sticks	4	<1	0.0	No	132	6.5	0.0	
Woolworths Original Thin Rice Crackers Minis	5	<1	0.0	No	86	2.5	1	
Woolworths Tasty Cheese & Crackers	9	<0.5	0.0	No	206	8.7	2	

Sweet Biscuits

Product Name	No. of Ingredients	Sugar (g)	Sugar (tsp)	Sugar in Top 3?	Sodium (mg)	Fat (g)	No. of Additives	Additives have potential effects?
Abe's Bagel Bites with Vegemite	33	1	0.3	No	120	1.5	8	
Arnott's Hundreds & Thousands	19	7.6	1.9	Yes	38	1.3	6	Yes
Arnott's Minis Chocolate Chip Cookies	16	7.4	1.9	Yes	73	6.3	4	
Arnott's Minis Scotch Finger Biscuits	11	4.8	1.2	Yes	120	5.3	2	
Arnott's Scotch Finger Santa's Biscuits	11	3.3	0.8	Yes	89	3.8	2	
Arnott's Snack Right Morning Slice Sultana	14	13.6	3.4	No	47	0.9	2	Yes
Arnott's Snack Right Pillow Wild Berry Flavour	28	15.7	3.9	No	66	2.5	8	Yes
Arnott's Tic Toc Biscuits	17	6.9	1.7	Yes	39	2.3	7	Yes

Product Name	No. of Ingredients	Sugar (g)	Sugar (tsp)	Sugar in Top 3?	Sodium (mg)	Fat (g)	No. of Additives	Additives have potential effects?
Arnott's Tiny Teddy Choc Chip	18	7	1.8	Yes	70	3.5	2	
Arnott's Tiny Teddy Chocolate	13	6.3	1.6	Yes	75	3.3	3	
Arnott's Tiny Teddy Honey	11	6.3	1.6	Yes	79	3.3	2	
Arnott's Tiny Teddy Oat & Honey	11	3.6	0.9	Yes	46	2.9	2	
Arnott's Wagon Wheels Original Minis	32	10.4	2.6	Yes	27	3.8	10	
Belmont Biscuit Co Choc Chip Teddy Tots	21	5.7	1.4	Yes	90	3.3	7	
Belmont Biscuit Co Choc Teddy Tots	18	6.2	1.6	Yes	88	3.3	8	
Belmont Biscuit Co Honey Teddy Tots	12	6.8	1.7	Yes	75	3.2	4	

Product Name	No. of Ingredients	Sugar (g)	Sugar (tsp)	Sugar in Top 3?	Sodium (mg)	Fat (g)	No. of Additives	Additives have potential effects?
Belmont Biscuit Co Hundreds & Thousands	27	7.1	1.8	Yes	66	4.7	13	Yes
Belmont Biscuit Co Hundreds & Thousands Teddy Tots	19	8	2.0	Yes	68	3	9	Yes
Belmont Biscuit Co Rice Entice Dark Chocolate	5	12.3	3.1	Yes	3	11.5	1	
Belmont Biscuit Co Rice Entice Milk Chocolate	8	15.9	4.0	Yes	34	10.9	2	
Belmont Biscuit Co Rice Entice Yogurt	9	17.1	4.3	Yes	31	11.8	2	
Belmont Biscuit Co Yogurt Fruit Bakes Strawberry Flavoured	41	15.5	3.9	No	92	3.6	10	Yes
Cadbury Oreo Cadbury Coated	15	16	4.0	Yes	98	4.3	5	
Cadbury Oreo Cadbury Coated Mint	19	16	4.0	Yes	99	8.1	8	

Product Name	No. of Ingredients	Sugar (g)	Sugar (tsp)	Sugar in Top 3?	Sodium (mg)	Fat (g)	No. of Additives	Additives have potential effects?
Mini Oreo Chocolate	12	8.7	2.2	Yes	122	4.7	5	
Nestle Starz DunkaRoos Choc Hazlenut Dip With Dunkaroos Biscuits	20	15.1	3.8	Yes	22	5.2	5	
Oreo Original Choc Cookie Sandwich with Sweet Vanilla Creme	12	11.2	2.8	Yes	154	6.1	5	
Oreo Wafer Sticks Milk Chocolate	20	5.1	1.3	Yes	18	3.7	8	
Paradise Uglies Multi Coloured Choc Chip	28	8	2.0	Yes	70	4.9	14	Yes
Unibic Anzac Biscuits Minis	12	8.1	2.0	Yes	50	5.2	2	
Woolworths Choc Chip Minis	22	7.5	1.9	Yes	60	5.4	5	
Woolworths Crème Wafer Minis	13	11.5	2.9	Yes	27	7.9	5	

Product Name	No. of Ingredients	Sugar (g)	Sugar (tsp)	Sugar in Top 3?	Sodium (mg)	Fat (g)	No. of Additives	Additives have potential effects?
Woolworths Hundreds & Thousands Biscuits	29	7.2	1.8	Yes	65	4.6	12	Yes
Woolworths Hundreds & Thousands White Choc Minis	24	7.6	1.9	Yes	63	4.8	9	Yes

Juice & Flavoured Milks

Product Name	No. of Ingredients	Sugar (g)	Sugar (tsp)	Sugar in Top 3?	Sodium (mg)	Fat (g)	No. of Additives	Additives have potential effects?
Berri Apple and Black-current Juice	6	25	6.3	No	20	<1	2	
Berri Apple Juice	4	25.3	6.3	No	20	<1	2	
Berri Orange Fruit Juice	4	20.8	5.2	No	20	<1	2	
Break Chocolate Milk	7	25.5	6.4	Yes	118	5	4	
Break Iced Coffee	4	24.3	6.1	Yes	118	4.8	1	
Coles Apple & Blackcur-rent Fruit Drink	8	27	6.8	No	13	<1	3	
Coles Apple & Blackcur-rent Juice	6	23.5	5.9	No	12	<1	3	
Coles Apple & Raspberry Fruit Drink	8	20.3	5.1	No	8	<1	4	

Product Name	No. of Ingredients	Sugar (g)	Sugar (tsp)	Sugar in Top 3?	Sodium (mg)	Fat (g)	No. of Additives	Additives have potential effects?
Coles Apple Fruit Drink	6	24	6.0	Yes	18	<1	2	
Coles Orange Fruit Drink	6	23.8	6.0	Yes	13	<1	2	
Coles Orange Juice	4	17	4.3	No	5	<1	2	
Devondale Moo Chocolate Milk	9	18.2	4.6	Yes	100	6.8	4	Yes
Devondale Moo Strawberry Milk	7	18.6	4.7	Yes	74	6.8	5	Yes
Farmdale Moo Box Strawberry Flavoured Milk	7	19	4.8	Yes	108	2	5	Yes
Golden Circle Apple Blackcurrent	7	24.9	6.2	No	2	0.0	2	
Golden Circle Apple Raspberry	7	24.9	6.2	No	3	0.0	2	

Product Name	No. of Ingredients	Sugar (g)	Sugar (tsp)	Sugar in Top 3?	Sodium (mg)	Fat (g)	No. of Additives	Additives have potential effects?
Golden Circle Fruit Juice Apple & Mango	4	21	5.3	No	6	0.2	1	
Golden Circle No Added Sugar Apple Mango Juice	4	24	6.0	No	2	0.2	1	
Golden Circle No Added Sugar Orange Juice	4	15.1	3.8	No	2	0.2	2	
Golden Circle No Added Sugar Tropical Juice	8	21.2	5.3	No	2	0.0	2	
Golden Circle Orange Burst	8	24.6	6.2	No	2	0.0	3	
Golden Circle Pine Orange	8	24.8	6.2	No	2	0.0	2	
Golden Circle Sunshine Punch	12	24.8	6.2	No	4	0.0	3	
Golden Circle Tropical Punch	11	24.8	6.2	No	3	0.0	3	

Product Name	No. of Ingredients	Sugar (g)	Sugar (tsp)	Sugar in Top 3?	Sodium (mg)	Fat (g)	No. of Additives	Additives have potential effects?
Golden Delicious Apple Splash	8	24.9	6.2	Yes	2	0.0	3	
Golden Delicious Golden Pash	9	24.8	6.2	No	3	0.0	3	
Golden Delicious Pineapple Burst	6	24.9	6.2	Yes	2	0.0	2	
Golden Delicious Summer Berries	9	24.9	6.2	No	1	0.0	2	
Just Juice Apple	4	20.2	5.1	No	16	<1	2	
Just Juice Apple Blackcurrent	5	20.2	5.1	No	16	<1	2	
Just Juice Orange	4	16.6	4.2	No	16	<1	2	
Just Juice Orange Mango	5	16.6	4.2	No	16	<1	2	

Product Name	No. of Ingredients	Sugar (g)	Sugar (tsp)	Sugar in Top 3?	Sodium (mg)	Fat (g)	No. of Additives	Additives have potential effects?
Just Juice Paradise Punch	9	20.2	5.1	No	16	<1	2	
Oak Chocolate Milk	13	30.5	7.6	Yes	128	5	6	Yes
Oak Strawberry Milk	7	31.3	7.8	Yes	110	8.3	3	Yes
Pop Tops Fruit Drink Apple	7	15	3.8	Yes	10	<1	4	Yes
Pop Tops Fruit Drink Apple Blackcurrent	9	14.8	3.7	No	10	<1	5	Yes
Pop Tops Fruit Drink Orange	9	13.8	3.5	Yes	8	0.0	6	Yes
Prima Apple Juice	5	17.8	4.5	Yes	16	0.0	2	
Prima Apple Watermelon Juice	6	17.8	4.5	No	16	0.0	2	

Product Name	No. of Ingredients	Sugar (g)	Sugar (tsp)	Sugar in Top 3?	Sodium (mg)	Fat (g)	No. of Additives	Additives have potential effects?
Prima Orange Juice	5	17.8	4.5	Yes	16	0.0	2	
Prima Orange Mango Juice	6	17.8	4.5	No	16	0.0	2	
Prima Tropical Juice	7	18	4.5	No	16	0.0	2	
Ribena Blackcurrent Fruit Drink	7	25.8	6.5	Yes	<5	<1	2	
Up&Go Chocolate	27	15.8	4.0	Yes	168	4.2	6	
Up&Go Strawberry	27	15.8	4.0	Yes	161	4.4	6	
Up&Go Vanilla Ice	27	15.8	4.0	Yes	158	4.3	6	
Westcliff Apple & Raspberry Fruit Drink	7	26	6.5	No	12	0.5	3	

Product Name	No. of Ingredients	Sugar (g)	Sugar (tsp)	Sugar in Top 3?	Sodium (mg)	Fat (g)	No. of Additives	Additives have potential effects?
Westcliff Apple Blackcurrent Juice	6	22.3	5.6	No	10	<0.3	3	
Westcliff Apple Juice	4	23.8	6.0	No	8	<0.3	2	
Westcliff Apple Juice Popper	6	27.5	6.9	No	18	0.5	4	Yes
Westcliff Orange Fruit Drink	6	23.3	5.8	Yes	13	0.2	3	
Westcliff Orange Juice	4	19.3	4.8	No	8	<0.3	2	
Westcliff Tropical Fruit Drink	9	28.8	7.2	No	13	0.2	3	
Woolworths Apple & Blackcurrent Juice	5	25	6.3	No	20	<1	2	
Woolworths Apple Fruit Drink	6	24.2	6.1	Yes	10	0.0	2	

Product Name	No. of Ingredients	Sugar (g)	Sugar (tsp)	Sugar in Top 3?	Sodium (mg)	Fat (g)	No. of Additives	Additives have potential effects?
Woolworths Apple Juice	4	25	6.3	No	20	<1	2	
Woolworths Orange Fruit Drink	6	24	6.0	Yes	10	0.0	2	
Woolworths Orange Juice	4	20.5	5.1	No	20	<1	2	
Woolworths Tropical Fruit Drink	8	24.2	6.1	Yes	10	0.0	2	

Yoghurt Tubs & Pouches

Product Name	No. of Ingredients	Sugar (g)	Sugar (tsp)	Sugar in Top 3?	Sodium (mg)	Fat (g)	No. of Additives	Additives have potential effects?
Brooklea Chocolate Stampede Dairy Snack	13	16.8	4.2	Yes	69	6.3	7	Yes
Brooklea Chocolate Stampede Dairy Snack Pouch	12	23.5	5.9	Yes	91	8.3	7	Yes
Brooklea Joi Deluxe Fruit Fantasy Yoghurt Mango	19	20	5.0	Yes	104	4.8	8	
Brooklea Joi Deluxe Fruit Fantasy Yoghurt Mixed Berry	22	19.7	4.9	Yes	105	5	7	
Brooklea Joi Deluxe Fruit Fantasy Yoghurt Strawberry	17	20.1	5.0	Yes	104	5	7	
Brooklea Les Petits Real Fruit Yoghurt Banana	14	13.2	3.3	Yes	46	2.9	7	
Brooklea Les Petits Real Fruit Yoghurt Strawberry	15	11.6	2.9	Yes	49	2.9	7	
Brooklea Les Petits Real Fruit Yoghurt Vanilla	11	12.5	3.1	Yes	48	2.9	5	

Product Name	No. of Ingredients	Sugar (g)	Sugar (tsp)	Sugar in Top 3?	Sodium (mg)	Fat (g)	No. of Additives	Additives have potential effects?
Brooklea Smooth Flavoured Yoghurt Family Pack Passionfruit	10	9.2	2.3	Yes	50	2.3	4	
Brooklea Smooth Flavoured Yoghurt Family Pack Strawberry	10	9.6	2.4	Yes	50	2.3	4	Yes
Brooklea Smooth Flavoured Yoghurt Family Pack Vanilla	11	9.2	2.3	Yes	50	2.3	5	
Brooklea Vanilla Custard Pouch	9	9	2.3	Yes	47	1.2	6	
Brooklea Yoghurt Squishy Banana	17	6	1.5	Yes	22	1.2	6	
Brooklea Yoghurt Squishy Blueberry	17	6.2	1.6	Yes	23	1.2	7	
Brooklea Yoghurt Squishy Strawberry	18	5.5	1.4	Yes	25	1.2	7	
Chobani Greek Yoghurt Banana Maple with Steel Cut Oats	12	16	4.0	No	32	0.7	3	Yes

Product Name	No. of Ingredients	Sugar (g)	Sugar (tsp)	Sugar in Top 3?	Sodium (mg)	Fat (g)	No. of Additives	Additives have potential effects?
Chobani Greek Yoghurt Mixed Berry with Steel Cut Oats & Ancient Grains	13	13.2	3.3	No	32	0.8	1	
Chobani Greek Yoghurt Strawberry	12	17.1	4.3	Yes	56	0.3	6	
Chobani Greek Yoghurt Vanilla	10	14.3	3.6	Yes	42	0.3	4	
Coles Banana & Passionfruit Fruit Puree Blend	5	9.9	2.5	No	16	0.5	2	
Coles Banana Yoghurt	17	6.8	1.7	Yes	24	1.5	5	
Coles Blueberry Yoghurt	16	8.4	2.1	No	29	1	6	
Coles Mango Fruit Puree Blend	5	11.3	2.8	Yes	12	0.5	2	
Coles Mixed Berry Fruit Puree Blend	5	10.6	2.7	Yes	<5	0.0	1	

Product Name	No. of Ingredients	Sugar (g)	Sugar (tsp)	Sugar in Top 3?	Sodium (mg)	Fat (g)	No. of Additives	Additives have potential effects?
Coles Strawberry Fruit Puree Blend	5	12	3.0	Yes	28	0.0	2	
Coles Strawberry Yoghurt	18	6.3	1.6	Yes	27	1.1	4	
Coles Vanilla Flavoured Yoghurt	15	5.7	1.4	Yes	27	1.2	4	
Coles Yoghurt Variety Pack Banana	15	12.4	3.1	Yes	32	2.9	7	
Coles Yoghurt Variety Pack Strawberry & Raspberry	15	11.3	2.8	Yes	35	3	6	Yes
Coles Yoghurt Variety Pack Vanilla	12	11.8	3.0	Yes	34	2.9	5	
Golden Circle Banana Berry Blast Apple Banana Strawberry & Raspberry	6	15.6	3.9	Yes	3	0.2	0.0	
Golden Circle Berry Buzz Apple, Blackcurrant, Blueberry & Raspberry Puree	6	14.6	3.7	Yes	5	0.4	0.0	

Product Name	No. of Ingredients	Sugar (g)	Sugar (tsp)	Sugar in Top 3?	Sodium (mg)	Fat (g)	No. of Additives	Additives have potential effects?
Golden Circle Passion Pulp Apple Passionfruit Puree	4	13.2	3.3	Yes	4	0.2	0.0	
Golden Circle Strawberry Squeeze Apple, Strawberry & Pear Puree	5	13.7	3.4	Yes	5	0.2	0.0	
Golden Circle Tropical Smash Apple, Pineapple & Banana Puree	5	22.9	5.7	Yes	5	0.2	0.0	
Goulburn Valley Fruit Plus Apple & Berry Enriched with Chia	8	14.9	3.7	No	17	0.7	2	
Goulburn Valley Fruit Plus Apple & Cinnamon Enriched with Chia	7	17.7	4.4	No	18	0.6	2	
Goulburn Valley Fruit Plus Apple, Banana & Honey Enriched with Coconut	9	17.3	4.3	No	20	3.6	2	
Goulburn Valley Fruit Plus Apple, Pineapple, Banana & Mango Enriched with Coconut	10	17.3	4.3	No	21	4.9	3	
Nestle Milo Energy Dairy Snack 12 pack 100g	21	13.2	3.3	Yes	65	4.4	4	

Product Name	No. of Ingredients	Sugar (g)	Sugar (tsp)	Sugar in Top 3?	Sodium (mg)	Fat (g)	No. of Additives	Additives have potential effects?
Nestle Milo Energy Dairy Snack 150g	23	19.8	5.0	No	98	6.6	4	
Paul's Banana Flavoured Yoghurt Finding Dory	14	8.4	2.1	Yes	43	2.9	7	
Paul's Chocolate Mousse Despicable Me	15	9.4	2.4	Yes	33	6	5	
Paul's Custard Snack Pack Vanilla	12	21.2	5.3	No	122	3.8	8	Yes
Paul's Milky Max Chocolate Custard	9	8.6	2.2	Yes	48	1.2	5	
Paul's Milky Max Chocolate Dairy Snack	12	17.7	4.4	Yes	72	6.1	7	Yes
Paul's Milky Max Vanilla Custard	9	9	2.3	Yes	47	1.2	6	
Paul's Strawberry Yoghurt Finding Dory	15	8.1	2.0	Yes	46	2.9	7	

Product Name	No. of Ingredients	Sugar (g)	Sugar (tsp)	Sugar in Top 3?	Sodium (mg)	Fat (g)	No. of Additives	Additives have potential effects?
Paul's Vanilla Yoghurt Finding Dory	12	8.4	2.1	Yes	43	2.9	5	
Petit Miam Apple & Blackcurrant Yoghurt Pouch	16	5.3	1.3	No	32	1.6	4	
Petit Miam Banana Yoghurt Pouch	16	5.2	1.3	No	30	1.6	6	
Petit Miam Blueberry Yoghurt Pouch	16	5.4	1.4	No	34	1.6	4	
Petit Miam Fruit Salad Yoghurt Pouch	19	5.2	1.3	No	31	1.6	6	
Petit Miam Strawberry Yoghurt Pouch	18	5.3	1.3	No	32	1.6	5	
Petit Miam Vanilla Yoghurt Pouch	14	5.3	1.3	No	31	1.6	5	
SPC Puree & Simple Apple & Banana	6	11.7	2.9	Yes	11	0.1	3	

Product Name	No. of Ingredients	Sugar (g)	Sugar (tsp)	Sugar in Top 3?	Sodium (mg)	Fat (g)	No. of Additives	Additives have potential effects?
SPC Puree & Simple Apple & Mango	6	11	2.8	Yes	10	0.1	3	
SPC Puree & Simple Apple & Mixed Berry	8	10.5	2.6	Yes	11	0.1	3	
SPC Puree & Simple Apple & Strawberry	7	10	2.5	Yes	11	0.1	3	
SPC Puree & Simple Apple, Peach & Pineapple	7	11	2.8	Yes	10	0.1	3	
Sweet Valley Spurtz Apple & Mixed Berry Fruit Puree	6	16.4	4.1	Yes	>5	>0.1	1	
Sweet Valley Spurtz Apple & Peach Fruit Puree	5	10.9	2.7	Yes	>5	0.5	2	
Sweet Valley Spurtz Apple & Strawberry Fruit Puree	5	14.7	3.7	Yes	>5	>0.1	1	
Tamar Valley Kids Blueberry Pouch	9	3.7	0.9	No	35	7.5	1	

Product Name	No. of Ingredients	Sugar (g)	Sugar (tsp)	Sugar in Top 3?	Sodium (mg)	Fat (g)	No. of Additives	Additives have potential effects?
Tamar Valley Kids Greek Yoghurt Strawberry	8	3.7	0.9	No	35	7.6	1	
Tamar Valley Kids Greek Yoghurt Vanilla	8	3.5	0.9	No	35	7.6	1	
Vaalia Probiotics Kids Yoghurt Strawberry	12	12.5	3.1	No	69	3.4	3	
Vaalia Probiotics Kids Yoghurt Vanilla	11	13.2	3.3	No	67	3.5	3	
Woolworths Banana Flavoured Custard	9	9.4	2.4	Yes	33	2.2	3	
Woolworths Banana Flavoured Yoghurt Pouch	17	6	1.5	Yes	24	1.4	5	
Woolworths Chocolate Flavoured Custard	9	9	2.3	Yes	33	2.4	2	
Woolworths Strawberry Flavoured Custard	8	9.3	2.3	Yes	33	2.3	3	Yes

Product Name	No. of Ingredients	Sugar (g)	Sugar (tsp)	Sugar in Top 3?	Sodium (mg)	Fat (g)	No. of Additives	Additives have potential effects?
Woolworths Strawberry Flavoured Yoghurt Pouch	16	6.6	1.7	Yes	26	1.3	6	
Woolworths Vanilla Flavoured Custard	7	8.9	2.2	Yes	31	2.2	2	
Woolworths Vanilla Flavoured Yoghurt Pouch	15	7.2	1.8	Yes	24	1.3	6	
YoGo Choc Rock	13	13	3.3	No	75	2.9	5	Yes
YoGo Mix (Choc Yogo & Choc Chips)	18	29.9	7.5	No	120	11.1	6	Yes
YoGo Mix (Choc Yogo & Mini M&Ms)	33	31.2	7.8	No	114	9	15	Yes
Yoplait Real Fruit Berry Punnet Raspberry	14	22.8	5.7	No	88	3.3	5	Yes
Yoplait Real Fruit Classics Mango	13	12.8	3.2	No	45	1.9	4	

Product Name	No. of Ingredients	Sugar (g)	Sugar (tsp)	Sugar in Top 3?	Sodium (mg)	Fat (g)	No. of Additives	Additives have potential effects?
Yoplait Real Fruit Classics Strawberry	15	12.5	3.1	No	49	1.9	6	
Yoplait Real Fruit Classics Vanilla	13	12.8	3.2	No	45	1.9	3	

Chocolate & Lollies

Product Name	No. of Ingredients	Sugar (g)	Sugar (tsp)	Sugar in Top 3?	Sodium (mg)	Fat (g)	No. of Additives	Additives have potential effects?
Allen's Snakes Alive	14	11	2.8	Yes	25	<1	2	
Choceur Chocolate Milk Sticks	14	8.8	2.2	Yes	20	6.9	2	
Choceur Cookie Milk Sticks	20	8.8	2.2	Yes	25	6.5	5	
Dominion Naturals Ropes	18	11.3	2.8	Yes	6	0.2	9	Yes
Dominion Naturals Ropes Animal Shapes	20	12.4	3.1	Yes	7	0.1	10	Yes
Dominion Naturals Ropes Sour Raspberry	14	11.4	2.9	Yes	11	0.1	7	Yes
Dominion Naturals Ropes Sporty Shapes	20	12.4	3.1	Yes	7	0.1	10	Yes
Dominion Naturals Ropes Strawberry, Raspberry & Blueberry	17	11.3	2.8	Yes	6	0.2	8	Yes

Product Name	No. of Ingredients	Sugar (g)	Sugar (tsp)	Sugar in Top 3?	Sodium (mg)	Fat (g)	No. of Additives	Additives have potential effects?
Dominion Naturals Ropes X + O's Shapes	17	12.4	3.1	Yes	7	0.1	8	Yes
Giant Value Bag Variety Mix Chocolates	22	9.1	2.3	Yes	20	3	8	Yes
Go Natural Berry Frugo's	17	19.2	4.8	Yes	14	7.6	5	Yes
Go Natural Twisters	10	11.5	2.9	No	1.4	<1	1	
Jurassic World Mixed Berry Flavoured Snacks	15	11.7	2.9	No	8	<1	5	Yes
Kinder Chocolate	12	6.7	1.7	Yes	15	4.4	1	
KitKat Chocolate	14	8.6	2.2	Yes	13	4.7	2	
Mamba Sour	10	2.1	0.5	Yes	<5	0.2	7	

Product Name	No. of Ingredients	Sugar (g)	Sugar (tsp)	Sugar in Top 3?	Sodium (mg)	Fat (g)	No. of Additives	Additives have potential effects?
MilkyWay Bars	12	7	1.8	Yes	8	1.8	1	
Nestle Smarties	19	9.1	2.3	Yes	6	2.4	9	Yes
Nice&Natural Fun Fruit Mix	15	8.8	2.2	Yes	9	<1	6	Yes
PJ Masks Fruit Tails Duos	17	11.7	2.9	No	8	<1	9	Yes
Skittles 12 fun bags	15	11	2.8	Yes	3	1	10	Yes
The Natural Confectionary Co. 25% Less Sugar Snakes	17	7.9	2.0	Yes	8	<1	2	
The Natural Confectionary Co. Snakes	16	11	2.8	Yes	6	<1	2	
Twix Chocolate	12	7.2	1.8	Yes	24	3.5	2	

Fruit & Jelly Cups

Product Name	No. of Ingredients	Sugar (g)	Sugar (tsp)	Sugar in Top 3?	Sodium (mg)	Fat (g)	No. of Additives	Additives have potential effects?
Coles Diced Peaches in Syrup	6	19	4.8	Yes	5	-	2	
Coles Fruit Salad in Syrup	8	17.5	4.4	No	4	0.2	2	
Coles Peach in Mango Flavoured Jelly	14	22.5	5.6	Yes	114	<1	10	
Coles Two Fruits in Strawberry Flavoured Jelly	16	22.5	5.6	No	114	<1	10	
SPC Mango Flavoured Jellly with Aussie Diced Peaches	11	14.2	3.6	No	49	0.1	7	
SPC Orange Flavoured Jelly with Diced Peaches	9	14.1	3.5	No	49	<0.1	7	
SPC Two Fruits in Juice	4	12.8	3.2	No	<5	<0.1	1	
Sweet Valley Apples in Pineapple Flavoured Jelly	14	22.5	5.6	Yes	46	<0.1	11	

Product Name	No. of Ingredients	Sugar (g)	Sugar (tsp)	Sugar in Top 3?	Sodium (mg)	Fat (g)	No. of Additives	Additives have potential effects?
Sweet Valley Diced Fruit Salad in Fruit Juice	6	16.3	4.1	No	2	<0.3	2	
Sweet Valley Diced Peaches in Fruit Juice	4	13.6	3.4	Yes	10	<0.1	2	
Sweet Valley Diced Two Fruits in Fruit Juice	5	13	3.3	Yes	8	<0.1	2	
Woolworths Apple in Pineapple Flavoured Jelly	14	21.6	5.4	Yes	44	<0.1	11	
Woolworths Peach in Strawberry Flavoured Jelly	14	21.2	5.3	Yes	45	<0.1	11	Yes
Woolworths Pear in Raspberry Flavoured Jelly	15	21	5.3	Yes	45	<0.1	12	Yes
Woolworths Two Fruits in Tropical Flavoured Jelly	16	21.1	5.3	Yes	45	<0.1	12	

Bread & Wraps

Product Name	No. of Ingredients	Sugar (g)	Sugar (tsp)	Sugar in Top 3?	Sodium (mg)	Fat (g)	No. of Additives	Additives have potential effects?
Abbott's Village Bakery Farmhouse Wholemeal	14	3	0.8	No	292	2.4	3	
Abbott's Village Bakery Grainy Wholemeal	21	2.9	0.7	No	319	3.8	3	
Abbott's Village Bakery Light Rye	16	2.1	0.5	No	274	2.3	3	
Abbott's Village Bakery Rustic White	14	3	0.8	No	282	2	3	
ALDI Specially Selected Brioche Burger Buns	18	5.5	1.375	No	230	4.2	3	
Australia's Own Organic Wraps With Quinoa	15	1.2	0.3	No	263	2.5	2	Yes
Bakers Life 14 Seeds Grains Sandwich Bread	25	1.3	0.325	No	296	6	0.0	
Bakers Life 85% Lower Carbs, Higher Protein Sandwich Bread	17	1.4	0.4	No	340	12.8	2	

Product Name	No. of Ingredients	Sugar (g)	Sugar (tsp)	Sugar in Top 3?	Sodium (mg)	Fat (g)	No. of Additives	Additives have potential effects?
Bakers Life Bagels	18	5.2	1.3	Yes	407	1.7	5	
Bakers Life Bakehouse Light Rye	15	1.9	0.5	No	304	1.6	1	
Bakers Life Bakehouse Mixed Grain	20	2.5	0.6	No	380	3.3	1	
Bakers Life Burger Rolls	18	4.5	1.1	No	260	6.2	5	
Bakers Life Cafe Style Raisin Loaf	16	12.5	3.125	No	176	2.3	2	
Bakers Life English Muffins	19	1.7	0.425	No	203	1.6	7	Yes
Bakers Life Grain Wise Sandwich	23	1.9	0.5	No	296	3	2	
Bakers Life Hot Dog Rolls	20	4.7	1.175	No	248	3.6	5	

Product Name	No. of Ingredients	Sugar (g)	Sugar (tsp)	Sugar in Top 3?	Sodium (mg)	Fat (g)	No. of Additives	Additives have potential effects?
Bakers Life Kornig Soy & Linseed Sandwich Bread	12	2.6	0.65	No	273	6.4	0.0	
Bakers Life Lebanese Bread Wholemeal	12	2.4	0.6	No	203	1.2	0.0	
Bakers Life Lebanese Flat Bread White	8	3.1	0.8	No	218	1	0.0	
Bakers Life Multi Grain Sandwich Bread	19	1.6	0.4	No	180	1.1	4	
Bakers Life Pane Di Casa	7	1.6	0.4	No	392	1.5	0.0	
Bakers Life Raisin Toast	18	11.9	2.975	No	189	2.5	2	
Bakers Life Sourdough Multi Grain	17	1.1	0.3	No	367	1.6	0.0	
Bakers Life Sourdough White	10	1.7	0.425	No	430	1.4	0.0	

Product Name	No. of Ingredients	Sugar (g)	Sugar (tsp)	Sugar in Top 3?	Sodium (mg)	Fat (g)	No. of Additives	Additives have potential effects?
Bakers Life Super Soft Flexible Wraps White	23	1.7	0.4	No	285	3.6	12	Yes
Bakers Life Super Soft Flexible Wraps Wholegrain	30	2.4	0.6	No	281	3.7	12	Yes
Bakers Life Super Soft Sandwich Loaf	15	1.9	0.5	No	198	1.2	2	
Bakers Life Turkish Bread Rolls	10	3.2	0.8	No	573	2	1	Yes
Bakers Life White Sandwich	17	1.9	0.5	No	225	1.2	4	
Casa Barelli Italian Style Pizza Bases	18	1.3	0.325	No	269	3.8	6	Yes
Coles Bakery Multigrain Toast Loaf	18	0.5	0.125	No	353	3.8	0.0	
Coles Bakery White Sandwich Loaf 680g	11	<1	0.0	No	214	1.2	1	

Product Name	No. of Ingredients	Sugar (g)	Sugar (tsp)	Sugar in Top 3?	Sodium (mg)	Fat (g)	No. of Additives	Additives have potential effects?
Coles Organic White Soft Wraps	12	2.1	0.5	No	225	2.9	2	
Coles White Soft Wraps	21	2.9	0.7	No	256	4	11	Yes
Coles Wholemeal & Grain Soft Wraps	30	2.3	0.6	No	256	4.2	11	Yes
Has No Gluten Free Seeded Sliced Bread	24	4.6	1.15	No	237	6.3	7	Yes
Has No Gluten Free White Sliced Bread	20	5	1.25	No	258	3	7	Yes
Helga's 5 Seeds Lower Carb	21	2	0.5	No	315	8.5	1	
Helga's Light Rye	15	2	0.5	No	300	1.7	1	
Helga's Mixed Grain	18	2.8	0.7	No	380	3	1	

Product Name	No. of Ingredients	Sugar (g)	Sugar (tsp)	Sugar in Top 3?	Sodium (mg)	Fat (g)	No. of Additives	Additives have potential effects?
Helga's Mixed Grain Mini Wraps	27	1.6	0.4	No	225	4.5	8	Yes
Helga's Pumpkin Seed & Grain	20	2.2	0.6	No	320	4.4	1	
Helga's Soy & Linseed	15	3	0.8	No	375	6	1	
Helga's Traditional White	14	2.5	0.6	No	335	2	1	
Helga's Traditional White Wraps	16	2.5	0.6	No	300	5.5	8	Yes
Helga's Traditional Wholemeal	14	2.5	0.6	No	335	2	1	
Helga's Wholegrain Wraps	23	2.2	0.6	No	315	6.2	8	Yes
Helga's Wholemeal & Seed Lower Carb	16	2	0.5	No	310	7.3	2	

Product Name	No. of Ingredients	Sugar (g)	Sugar (tsp)	Sugar in Top 3?	Sodium (mg)	Fat (g)	No. of Additives	Additives have potential effects?
Helga's Wholemeal Grain	19	3.3	0.8	No	375	3.8	1	
Mission Soft Wraps Wholegrain	30	2	0.5	No	639	6.8	9	Yes
Mission Super Soft Wholewheat Mini Wraps	16	1.2	0.3	No	418	4.5	9	Yes
Mission Super Soft Wraps Lite	16	2.3	0.6	No	669	2.1	9	Yes
Mountain Bread Natural Wraps	4	0.5	0.1	No	100	0.4	0.0	
Mountain Bread Rice Wraps	6	0.4	0.1	No	98	0.3	0.0	
Mountain Bread Rye Wraps	6	0.5	0.1	No	100	0.4	0.0	
Tiptop 9 Grain Original	26	1.6	0.4	No	296	3.7	3	

Product Name	No. of Ingredients	Sugar (g)	Sugar (tsp)	Sugar in Top 3?	Sodium (mg)	Fat (g)	No. of Additives	Additives have potential effects?
Tiptop Sunblest Soft White Sandwich	13	1.8	0.5	No	296	1.5	3	
Viva Plus Wholemeal Smooth Sandwich Bread	21	1.9	0.5	No	296	1.9	2	
Woolworths Essential White Sandwich	12	2	0.5	No	264	1.6	2	
Woolworths Extra Soft White Loaf	10	0.8	0.2	No	234	2	0.0	
Woolworths Soft Multi-grain Sandwich	15	1.6	0.4	No	264	2	2	
Woolworths Soft White Toast	13	2.3	0.575	No	312	2.3	2	
Woolworths Soft Wholemeal Sandwich	13	1.6	0.4	No	264	2.3	2	
Woolworths Soft Wraps White	17	1.1	0.3	No	154	3.7	7	Yes
Woolworths Soft Wraps Wholegrain	31	1.2	0.3	No	158	2.4	7	Yes

Appendix 2
Other Names for Sugar

Processed food relies on what is called the bliss point. It's the right combination of sugar, salt and fat that creates the optimum deliciousness. Adding sugar or a sugar alternative has become a big way manufacturers achieve the bliss point.

Thanks to the incredible work of people like Sarah Wilson previously from I Quit Sugar, David Gillespie, author of Sweet Poison, Damon Gameau from That Sugar Movement and consumer group Choice, more people have become aware of sugar and the issues it's having on our health.

However, on the flip side to all this new awareness that's been raised about sugar is manufacturers ability to reformulate their products to produce the sweet taste by using ingredients which no longer use the word sugar. For unsuspecting consumers, they may not realise some of the ingredients are just another way of saying sugar.

With the permission from That Sugar Movement, we include this picture from their wonderful website and their books (a must get) that outlines 60 different names for sugar. Start looking out for these in the ingredients.

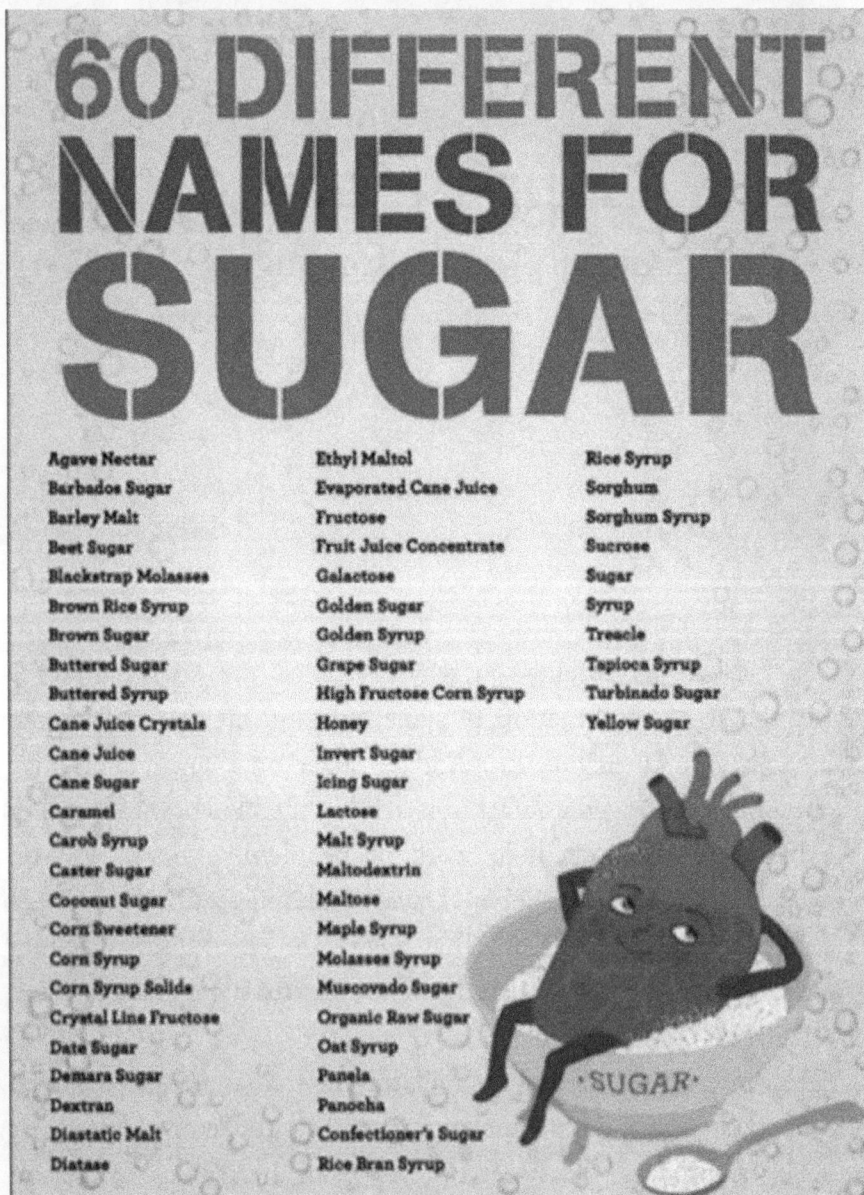

60 DIFFERENT NAMES FOR SUGAR

Agave Nectar	Ethyl Maltol	Rice Syrup
Barbados Sugar	Evaporated Cane Juice	Sorghum
Barley Malt	Fructose	Sorghum Syrup
Beet Sugar	Fruit Juice Concentrate	Sucrose
Blackstrap Molasses	Galactose	Sugar
Brown Rice Syrup	Golden Sugar	Syrup
Brown Sugar	Golden Syrup	Treacle
Buttered Sugar	Grape Sugar	Tapioca Syrup
Buttered Syrup	High Fructose Corn Syrup	Turbinado Sugar
Cane Juice Crystals	Honey	Yellow Sugar
Cane Juice	Invert Sugar	
Cane Sugar	Icing Sugar	
Caramel	Lactose	
Carob Syrup	Malt Syrup	
Caster Sugar	Maltodextrin	
Coconut Sugar	Maltose	
Corn Sweetener	Maple Syrup	
Corn Syrup	Molasses Syrup	
Corn Syrup Solids	Muscovado Sugar	
Crystal Line Fructose	Organic Raw Sugar	
Date Sugar	Oat Syrup	
Demara Sugar	Panela	
Dextran	Panocha	
Diastatic Malt	Confectioner's Sugar	
Diatase	Rice Bran Syrup	

·SUGAR·

Image from That Sugar Movement

Appendix 3
Names of MSG Equivalents

In Chapters 5 & 6 Francine Bell from Additive Free Kids shared why looking out for MSG is so important. If you haven't read that, please be sure to go back to it but in short, some processed foods would be very bland if it wasn't for a flavour enhancer. MSG is a flavour enhancer.

Please check out the great work of Sue Dengate and her food scientist husband, Dr Howard Dengate, over at The Food Intolerance Network. Their website is loaded with information about MSG and other additives, and they have graciously granted us permission to use the table and information below.

The information contained here has been summarised from The Food Intolerance website fedup.com.au. [70]

One word (10 ways)	620, 621, 622, 623, 624, 625, Flavour*, HPP, HVP, Yeast* (not baker's yeast)
Two words (36 ways)	Ammonium glutamate, BBQ flavour, Calcium glutamate , Cheese powder, Corn protein*, Flavour (gluten), Glutamic acid, Hydrolysed casein, Hydrolysed corn, Hydrolysed maize, Hydrolysed protein, Hydrolysed rice, Hydrolysed soy, Hydrolysed vegetable, Hydrolysed wheat, Hydrolysed yeast, Kelp extract, Magnesium glutamate, Maize protein*, Miso powder, Monoammonium glutamate, Monopotassium glutamate, Monosodium glutamate, Natural flavour*, Nutritional yeast, Plant protein*, Potassium glutamate, Rice protein*, Savoury yeast, Soy protein*, Soy sauce, Umami flavour, Vegetable extract, Vegetable protein*, Wheat protein*, Yeast extract.
Three words (63 ways)	Autolysed yeast extract, Natural flavour soy, Nutritional yeast extract, Savoury yeast flakes, Soy sauce powder, Vegetable extract (maize), Vegetable extract (soy), Vegetable extract (wheat), Yeast extract powder; plus any combination of the words below in groups of 3: Autolysed, Hydrolysed, or Lyophilised with Casein, Corn, Maize, Plant, Rice, Soy, Vegetable, Wheat, or Yeast with Extract or Protein eg Hydrolysed rice extract.

Four words (20 ways)	Dehydrated vegetable seasoning (corn), Dehydrated vegetable seasoning (maize), Dehydrated vegetable seasoning (rice), Dehydrated vegetable seasoning (soy), Dehydrated vegetable seasoning (wheat), Flavour natural (contains corn), Flavour natural (contains maize), Flavour natural (contains rice), Flavour natural (contains soy), Flavour natural (contains wheat), Plant protein extract (corn), Plant protein extract (maize), Plant protein extract (rice), Plant protein extract (soy), Plant protein extract (wheat), Vegetable protein extract (corn), Vegetable protein extract (maize), Vegetable protein extract (rice), Vegetable protein extract (soy), Vegetable protein extract (wheat).

Appendix 4
Other Links

Below are some links you may find useful.

Finding Quality Suppliers

- Australian Farmers Market Association – find a Farmers Market
  https://farmersmarkets.org.au/find-a-market/
- The Wholefood Collective for pantry staples
  https://thewholefoodcollective.com.au/?ref=22
- Bulk Food Directory
  https://sustainabletable.org.au/all-things-ethical-eating/bulk-food-directory/
- Additive Free Marketplace
  https://www.additivefreemarketplace.com.au/

Food Additives/Sugar/Labelling

- Additive Free Kids with Francine Bell
  https://www.additivefreekids.com.au/
- Food Intolerance Network – Dr Howard Dengate and Sue Dengate
  https://fedup.com.au/
- Additive Free Lifestyle – Australian Sisters Tracy and Jo
  https://additivefreelifestyle.com/
- That Sugar Movement – Australian Damon Gameau and team
  https://thatsugarmovement.com/
- Choice – Australia's leading consumer advocacy group
  https://www.choice.com.au/
- Foodwatch – with Australian Nutritionist Catherine Saxby
  https://www.foodwatch.com.au

Wellness Websites I trust

There are seriously so many ways to educate yourself about food these days. In addition to the links above, I have listed some other wellness websites I trust.

- Food Matters TV – think Netflix but for health – loaded with inspirational films, guided programs, meal plans and more. We love our FMTV membership.
  https://fmtv.com
- Well Nourished – with Australian Naturopath Georgia Harding – incredibly simple wellness articles and delicious recipes.
  https://wellnourished.com.au/ref/23/
- Jo Atkinson – Australian Nutritionist (and contributor to this book) – well written and simple to read health articles, especially around gut health
  https://www.joatkinson.com.au/

- Changing Habits – led by Cyndi O'Meara, one of Australia's leading nutritionist, film maker, author. Incredible articles, loads of free recipes and a wholefoods store too. **https://changinghabits.com.au/**
- Low Tox Life – with Australia's Alexx Stuart, author and change maker. Inspirational articles about toxins in food and your surroundings and awesome recipes. **https://www.lowtoxlife.com/**

Online Stores for Lunchbox and Products to Reduce Your Environmental Foot Print

- Sustainahome - sustainable living products at your fingertips. Packet free lunchbox tools and products for around the home **https://sustainahome.com/**
- Biome **http://rootcau.se/biome**
- Munchbox **https://www.mymunchbox.com.au**

Specialists to Help with Fussy Eating/ Sensory / Gut Issues etc

These are some people I met in our travels and I love their approach. Reach out for support.

- Jo Atkinson – Nutritionist Specialist **https://www.joatkinson.com.au/**
- Let's Eat Paediatric Speech Pathology – Val Gent. **https://www.letseatspeech.com.au/**
- Justine Moore – Nourishing Love Nutrition – GAPS Practioner **http://nourishinglove.com.au/**

- Little Fusspots - Beth Bonfiglio
  https://www.littlefusspot.com/
- Natural Super Kids – Naturopath Jessica Donovan
  https://naturalsuperkids.com/

Endnotes

1. The Root Cause – Real Food Lunchbox Project Preliminary Report August 2018 – https://www.dropbox.com/s/90n5a9vta6uxvom/The-Real-Food-Lunchbox-Project-Preliminary-Report-w-Images-20180806.pdf?dl=0

2. Senator Lisa Singh – Obesity In Australia Inquiry Report Speech – https://www.youtube.com/watch?v=3hFnl7iASMc&feature=youtu.be&t=215

3. National Health Study: First Results, 2017-2018 – https://www.abs.gov.au/ausstats/abs@.nsf/mf/4364.0.55.001

4. National Health Study: First Results, 2017-2018 – https://www.abs.gov.au/ausstats/abs@.nsf/mf/4364.0.55.001

5. The Mental Health of Children & Adolescents 2015 – https://www1.health.gov.au/internet/main/publishing.nsf/Content/9DA8CA21306FE6EDCA257E2700016945/$File/pt2.pdf

6. The Mental Health of Children & Adolescents 2015 – https://www1.health.gov.au/internet/main/publishing.nsf/Content/9DA8CA21306FE6EDCA257E2700016945/$File/pt2.pdf

7. The Mental Health of Children & Adolescents 2015 – https://www1.health.gov.au/internet/main/publishing.nsf/Content/9DA8CA21306FE6EDCA257E2700016945/$File/pt2.pdf

8. Learning Difficulties Australia – https://www.ldaustralia.org/302.html

9. Autism Prevalence in Australia 2015 – http://a4.org.au/prevalence2015

10. Global Asthma Report 2018 – http://www.globalasthmareport.org/burden/burden.php

11. AIWH Type 2 Diabetes in Australia's children and young people 2014 – https://www.aihw.gov.au/reports/diabetes/type-2-diabetes-in-australia-s-children-and-young/contents/table-of-contents

12. ABC Science News – Food Allergies are all too common in Australia 12 Feb 2019 – https://www.abc.net.au/news/science/2019-02-12/what-can-be-done-about-food-allergy-increases-in-australia/10799390

13. National Health Study: First Results, 2017-2018 – https://www.abs.gov.au/ausstats/abs@.nsf/mf/4364.0.55.001

14. Australian Institute of Health & Welfare (AIHW) Nutrition Across The Life Stages Report 2018 – https://www.aihw.gov.au/reports/food-nutrition/nutrition-across-the-life-stages/contents/summary

15. Australian Institute of Health & Welfare (AIHW) Nutrition Across The Life Stages Report 2018 – https://www.aihw.gov.au/reports/food-nutrition/nutrition-across-the-life-stages/contents/summary

16. DAA Media Release 18/5/2017 – https://www.dropbox.com/s/ev5yucig2t2rny5/Aussie-spending-the-majority-of-food-budget-on-junk-food-FINAL.pdf?dl=0

17. InsightPlus Research 19 August 2019 – https://insightplus.mja.com.au/2019/32/screen-time-in-under-2s-breathtaking/

18. DAA Media Release 18/5/2017 – https://www.dropbox.com/s/ev5yucig2t2rny5/Aussie-spending-the-majority-of-food-budget-on-junk-food-FINAL.pdf?dl=0

19. Prevalence of Cardiovascular Disease Factors Among US Adolescents – Paediatrics June 2012, Volume 129 – https://pediatrics.aappublications.org/content/129/6/1035.short

20. Supermarket Sales Tricks – Choice – https://www.choice.com.au/shopping/everyday-shopping/supermarkets/articles/supermarket-sales-tricks

21. Behaviour and Discipline in Schools – The Food For Life Partnership (UK) – https://publications.parliament.uk/pa/cm201011/cmselect/cmeduc/writev/behaviour/we23.htm

22. Association of Symptoms of Attention-Deficit/Hyperactivity Disorder with Physical Activity, Media Time, and Food Intake in Children and Adolescents – https://www.ncbi.nlm.nih.gov/pmc/articles/PMC3498177/

23. What is the Relationship Between Child Nutrition and School Outcomes? – https://www.researchgate.net/publication/252059240_What_is_the_relationship_between_child_nutrition_and_school_outcomes

24. Nutrition and Academic Performance in School-Age Children The Relation to Obesity and Food Insufficiency – https://www.longdom.org/open-access/nutrition-and-academic-performance-in-school-age-children-the-relation-to-obesity-and-food-insufficiency-2155-9600.1000190.pdf

25. New York City Public Schools – Four Years of Success – https://www.dropbox.com/s/1sh4kwh0ixs2ond/NewYorkCityPublicSchools_SchoolFoodStudy.pdf?dl=0

26. The Root Cause Food & Waste Report – Overall Dashboard November 2019

27. The Five Food Groups – Eat For Health.gov.au – https://www.eatforhealth.gov.au/food-essentials/five-food-groups

28. World Nutrition Volume 7, Number 1-3, January-March 2016 The Food System – Food Classification – https://archive.wphna.org/wp-content/uploads/2016/01/WN-2016-7-1-3-28-38-Monteiro-Cannon-Levy-et-al-NOVA.pdf

29. World Nutrition Volume 7, Number 1-3, January-March 2016 The Food System – Food Classification – https://archive.wphna.org/wp-content/uploads/2016/01/WN-2016-7-1-3-28-38-Monteiro-Cannon-Levy-et-al-NOVA.pdf

30. Michael Pollan's Talk – How Cooking Can Change Your Life – https://www.youtube.com/watch?v=TX7kwfE3cJQ

31. New Analysis by The George Institute For Global Health – https://www.georgeinstitute.org/media-releases/australias-supermarket-shelves-full-of-highly-processed-and-highly-unhealthy-foods

32. Overview of Food Ingredients, Additives & Colors – U.S. Food & Drug Administration – https://www.fda.gov/food/food-ingredients-packaging/overview-food-ingredients-additives-colors

33. Chemical preservatives impact food security – Poughkeepsie journal, Feb 18, 2016 – https://www.poughkeepsiejournal.com/story/life/2016/02/18/earth-wise-chemical-preservatives/80555070/

34. IARC Review Consumption of Red Meat and Processed Meat – https://www.iarc.fr/wp-content/uploads/2018/07/pr240_E.pdf

35. Additive Free Marketplace Directory – https://www.additivefreemarketplace.com.au/

36. List of Aspartame Products – http://www.drugsdb.com/cib/aspartame/list-of-aspartame-products

37. Metabolic Syndrome – Mayo Clinic – https://www.mayoclinic.org/diseases-conditions/metabolic-syndrome/symptoms-causes/syc-20351916

38. Skipping Breakfast on the Rise Among Aussie Children – https://www.cereal4brekkie.org.au/skipping-breakfast-on-the-rise-among-aussie-school-children/

39. Foodbank Finds Aussie Schools Kids Missing Most Important Meal of the Day – https://www.foodbank.org.au/wp-content/uploads/2019/05/Foodbank-Hunger-in-the-Classroom-Report-May-2015.pdf

40. Evaluation of the School Breakfast Clubs Program – Interim Report – https://www.foodbankvictoria.org.au/wp-content/blogs.dir/18/files/2018/04/School-Breakfast-Club-2018-Interim-Report.pdf

41. Breakfast Cereal Consumption in Australia 2014 – https://www.cereal4brekkie.org.au/wp-content/uploads/2014/11/Breakfast-Cereal-Consumption-in-Australia.pdf

42. Choice – Breakfast Cereals Review – https://www.choice.com.au/food-and-drink/bread-cereal-and-grains/cereal-and-muesli/articles/breakfast-cereal-review

43. Early Lunch Curbs Unruly Schoolyard Behaviour – The Advertiser, Adelaide Oct 20, 2012 – https://www.adelaidenow.com.au/news/south-australia/early-lunch-curbs-unruly-schoolyard-behaviour/news-story/b182f6f7e23720d841301f719d242e4f

44. Qualitative Investigation of Barriers and Facilitators Into the Adoption of Crunch n Sip Program in WA Primary Schools – https://www.crunchandsip.com.au/assets/downloads/2012-04-10-cbrcc-crunchsip-evaluation.pdf

45. ABC – Food For Thought, Episode 1 – http://abccommercial.com/librarysales/program/food-thought

46. KESAB Environmental Solutions Data over 10 year period 2006-2016 – https://www.dropbox.com/s/tg64qm8z71776pz/2016_ave_results_for_sa_primary_schools.pdf?dl=0

47. The Root Cause Overall Food & Waste Benchmark Report – Nov 2019

48. NOTED – An Otara Primary School Bans Sugary Drinks – And Sees Immediate Benefits. 6 May 2017 – https://www.noted.co.nz/health/health/an-otara-primary-school-bans-sugary-drinks-and-sees-immediate-benefits/

49. Nutrition Program at Outback Queensland School Helps Entire Community – https://www.abc.net.au/news/2017-03-13/nutrition-program-at-outback-queensland-school-changes-community/8275524

50. National Health Study: First Results, 2017-2018 – https://www.abs.gov.au/ausstats/abs@.nsf/mf/4364.0.55.001

51. Australian Institute of Health & Welfare (AIHW) Nutrition Across The Life Stages Report 2018 – https://www.aihw.gov.au/reports/food-nutrition/nutrition-across-the-life-stages/contents/table-of-contents

52. Today Report - Food Q&A - Just what is natural flavouring? – https://www.today.com/food/food-q-just-what-natural-flavoring-2D80554450

53. How The Food Industry Helps Engineer Our Cravings – https://www.npr.org/sections/thesalt/2015/12/16/459981099/how-the-food-industry-helps-engineer-our-cravings

54. That Sugar Movement – Sugar in Seemingly Healthy Foods – https://thatsugarmovement.com/sugar-in-seemingly-healthy-foods/

55. That Sugar Movement – https://thatsugarmovement.com/how-much-sugar-should-i-eat/

56. The Science Behind the Sweetness in Our Diets – Bulletin of The World Health Organisation – https://www.who.int/bulletin/volumes/92/11/14-031114.pdf

57. That Sugar Movement – What's the Added Sugar Limit for Kids? – https://thatsugarmovement.com/whats-the-added-sugar-limit-for-kids/

58. That Sugar Movement – **https://thatsugarmovement.com/** – and Sugars Intake for Adults & Children Guideline – WHO – **https://www. who.int/nutrition/publications/guidelines/sugars_intake/en/**

59. Nutrition across life stages, Summary, Australian Institute of Health and Welfare - **https://www.aihw.gov.au/reports/ food-nutrition/ nutrition-across-the-life-stages/contents/ summary ?fbclid=IwAR125Hddj6osuwkQkQgq PRTBf6HohzK10dW07X5KNuB4Qj4_RaO458sGKmY**

60. National Health Study : First Results, 2017-2018 – **https://www. abs.gov.au/ausstats/abs@.nsf/mf/4364.0.55.001**

61. The George Institute – Australian Salt Intake Twice the WHO Recommended Level – **https://www.georgeinstitute.org.au/media-releases/australian-salt-intake-twice-the-who-recommended-level**

62. Catherine Saxelby Food Watch – How to Covert Sodium to Salt and Salt to Sodium – **https://foodwatch.com.au/blog/measures-and-conversions/item/how-to-convert-sodium-to-salt-and-salt-to-sodium.html**

63. Aussie Kids Are Eating Alarming Levels of Salt – **https://www. georgeinstitute.org.au/media-releases/aussie-kids-are-eating-alarming-levels-of-salt**

64. Aussie Kids Are Eating Alarming Levels of Salt – **https://www. georgeinstitute.org.au/media-releases/aussie-kids-are-eating-alarming-levels-of-salt**

65. World Health Organisation – Healthy Diet – **https://www.who.int/ news-room/fact-sheets/detail/healthy-diet**

66. Amen Clinics – Why Are 'Healthy Fats' So Important? – January 11 2018 – **https://www.amenclinics.com/blog/why-healthy-fats-are-important/**

67. Mind Body Green – If You're Going to Eat One Thing Daily For Your Brain Health, This Should Be It. Dr Mark Hyman – **https://www. mindbodygreen.com/articles/how-healthy-fats-benefit-brain-health**

68. Changing Habits – Why I Never Consume Vegetable Oils – **https:// changinghabits.com.au/blog/2016/03/22/why-i-never-consume-vegetable-oils/**

69. University Health News – Omega 6 –v– Omega 3 Fatty Acids: What You Should Know – **https://universityhealthnews.com/daily/nutrition/omega-6-vs-omega-3-fatty-acids/**

70. Food Intolerance Network – 129 Ways to Add MSG to Fool Consumers – **https://www.fedup.com.au/news/blog/129-ways-to-add-msg-and-fool-consumers**